Borderline Personality Disorder

Borderline Personality Disorder
A practical guide to treatment

Roy Krawitz
*Consultant Psychiatrist to the area of borderline
personality disorder,
Health Waikato,
Hamilton,
New Zealand*

Christine Watson
*Director,
Spectrum,
The Personality Disorder Service for Victoria,
Melbourne,
Australia*

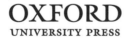
OXFORD
UNIVERSITY PRESS

OXFORD
UNIVERSITY PRESS

Great Clarendon Street, Oxford OX2 6DP

Oxford University Press is a department of the University of Oxford.
It furthers the University's objective of excellence in research, scholarship, and
education by publishing worldwide in

Oxford New York
Auckland Bangkok Buenos Aires Cape Town Chennai Dar es Salaam
Delhi Hong Kong Istanbul Karachi Kolkata Kuala Lumpur Madrid
Melbourne Mexico City Mumbai Nairobi São Paulo Shanghai
Taipei Tokyo Toronto

Oxford is a registered trade mark of Oxford University Press in the UK and in
certain other countries

Published in the United States
by Oxford University Press Inc., New York

© Oxford University Press 2003

The moral rights of the author have been asserted

Database right Oxford University Press (maker)

First published 2003
Reprinted 2004

A catalogue record for this book is available from the British Library

ISBN 0 19 852067 0

10 9 8 7 6 5 4 3 2

Typeset by Cepha Imaging Private Ltd.
Printed in Great Britain
on acid-free paper by Biddles Ltd, King's Lynn, Norfolk

Preface

The book focuses on work in adult mental health services, and does not attempt to cover specialist areas (e.g. child, adolescent and forensic services) or work with indigenous populations. Gender and sexual abuse issues are important, as 75% of people meeting diagnostic criteria for borderline personality disorder are female and 70% have a history of sexual abuse. These issues, whilst commented on, have not been comprehensively addressed in this book as there are ongoing forums available where they have been and will continue to be explored.

R.K.
C.W.
January 2003

Acknowledgements

Thanks to clients, colleagues, supervisees, and workshop participants for the knowledge and opportunities for learning they have provided. Thanks to the American Psychiatric Association for their permission to reprint the DSM-IV diagnostic criteria for borderline personality disorder and the Williams quote, Balance Program for providing the template on which the "Fictitious Example of a Crisis Plan" is based, Canadian Family Physician for permission to reprint the vignette "Molly", the Center for Psychiatric Rehabilitation for permission to reprint the item by Everett and Nelson, the Cutting Edge for permission to quote from their newsletter, Guilford Press for permission to reprint quotations from Rockland, Beck/Freeman & Associates, Leibenluft, Gardner and Cowdry, and Linehan, Jackson for permission to use several quotations, the Mental Health Commission for permission to reprint the section "Clinician values and feelings", and Williams for permission to adapt and print the exercise "Self-exploration of reasons for self-harm".

Contents

Part 3 Stigma, language, clinician feelings, and resourcing

Part 4 The legal environment

Terminology

The term "borderline personality disorder" is experienced as offensive and unhelpful by many. Whilst more meaningful and useful terminology is explored, it seemed best to use a term that will be clearly understood by readers. The phrase "people meeting diagnostic criteria for borderline personality disorder", whilst a mouthful, is used to highlight the above issues. The terminology "case management" which is frequently offensive to clients is used because it is also clearly understood by readers.

Abbreviations

Diagnostic and Statistical Manual of Mental Disorders, Fourth Edition is abbreviated throughout as DSM-IV.

Dialectical behavior therapy is abbreviated throughout as DBT.

Posttraumatic stress disorder is abbreviated throughout as PTSD.

Molly

"Molly suffered repeated severe physical, sexual and emotional abuse at the hands of several family members throughout her childhood and adolescence. Even as a young adult, she remained at risk whenever she had any contact with her family. She was removed from the care of her parents several times during childhood, but on each occasion was eventually returned to their care. Frustrated, ashamed, and convinced that she was responsible for all the problems in her family, Molly began to hit herself with belts, cords and sticks when she was 12 years old. She described how she learned "cutting" from another patient while in a psychiatric hospital. By the time we met, she had a history of more than 50 overdoses, using medications prescribed by different physicians as well as those available over the counter. She had added burning her limbs and alcohol abuse to her repertoire of self-injury. None of this self-abuse caused physical pain, but each episode was temporarily effective in relieving her frustration. Massively obese, constantly starving and overeating, she spent more time in hospital than in the community. No treatment programs helped; borderline personality disorder was diagnosed, and she began to feel and fear the inevitable rejection of her caretakers" (Haswell and Graham, 1996).

(Reproduced with permission from Canadian Family Physician)

Introduction

Gina, a community mental health nurse, is allocated to see Anne, a client, at a routine referral meeting. Gina planned to maintain regular contact with Anne and "keep an eye on her" whilst Anne was on the waiting list to see one of the people ascribed skill in treating people such as Anne. Anne had been previously diagnosed as meeting diagnostic criteria for borderline personality disorder. She had been attending psychiatric services for eight years which included 20 admissions to acute psychiatric units and a similar number of visits to emergency departments as a result of self-harm. Anne self-harmed most weeks, sometimes in a manner which was like "playing Russian roulette".

Gina did not see herself as being especially skilful in the treatment of people meeting diagnostic criteria for borderline personality disorder but she knew she had attained professional maturity in her practice as a psychiatric nurse. She was compassionate and believed that people meeting diagnostic criteria for borderline personality disorder were deserving of treatment and could get better. Unlike many of her colleagues, she had maintained optimism and enthusiasm for her work and her clients.

Gina met Anne and together over a period of storms, crises, emergency service and acute inpatient admissions, they collaboratively developed a clinical plan including acute admission and crisis plans. Michael and Dorothy worked on the crisis and acute inpatient teams and did not see themselves as having specific expertise in this area but, like Gina, did have considerable general mental health skills. There were discussions between Gina, Michael, Dorothy and Anne with significant conflicts of views. Over the months however, they developed a coherent plan they could agree to, for the most part.

One year after treatment with Gina had begun, improvements were clearly noticeable. In the previous six months, Anne had been admitted to hospital on only one occasion, for a pre-agreed 48-hour period. Anne's self-harm episodes were a quarter of what they had been and the severity of self-harm was no longer life endangering. Contact with the crisis service was earlier in the crisis spiral and crises took less time to resolve. Crisis team staff began to quite like Anne and no longer saw her as a burden.

This book is written for people like Gina, Michael and Dorothy who have natural talents and use and modify skills they have developed in their general mental health work. The book provides a pragmatic, down-to-earth treatment approach using existing mental health workforce skills as a base of knowledge to draw from and build on.

Skilled psychotherapists can use the principles of the book in working alongside generalist clinicians and to assist development of organizational structures and responses likely to enhance client outcome. Having therapists skilled in specific therapies (especially those studied and researched in this area) is an important and synergistic endeavour, alongside the development of skills across the whole of mental health services.

The fictitious clinical vignettes found throughout the text are intended, for interested readers, as catalysts for thought and discussion of the topics covered. This may include general principles guiding effective treatment and specifically what is required in the clinical situation outlined.

There is a paucity of evidence-based research The limited evidence-based research is highlighted, along with international opinion of best practice and accounts of client and clinician experience. Gaps in knowledge are also identified. This book is a synthesis and distillation of current and emerging opinion, thought and practice. Readers who are interested may wish to examine the American Psychiatric Association's guidelines (American Psychiatric Association 2001) and the concerns the guidelines raise amongst commentators (Paris 2002; Sanderson, Swenson and Bohus 2002; Tyrer 2002).

Part 1

Background to treatment

Origins of the label "borderline personality disorder"

The term "borderline personality disorder" arose out of the experiences of psychoanalysts. They identified a cluster of clients who responded differently in treatment to clients categorised at the time as "neurotic" or "psychotic". The presentation was initially similar to those who were "neurotic" but response to treatment was very different. The term "borderline" referred to the belief that these people were on the "border" between neurosis and psychosis. Whilst some clients do have psychotic or psychotic-like experiences, the notion that clients meeting diagnostic criteria for borderline personality disorder are on the border between neurosis and psychosis is no longer held.

The response to the name "borderline personality disorder" has been largely negative, although not entirely so. Some clients when provided with the term and the DSM-IV criteria have found it a positive experience; "Yes, this fits" and "professionals understand". However, most people are unhappy with the term. Many clinicians see it as lacking validity and reliability. Many clients perceive the term "personality disorder" as disrespectful, blaming and attacking their very deepest being. Because of the pejorative way that people meeting diagnostic criteria for borderline personality disorder are frequently seen, the term has attracted further disrepute. This probably would have occurred with any term used and is likely to become attached to any alternative term, unless attitudes change.

Out of the disquiet with the term "borderline personality disorder" and with an awareness of the frequent history of trauma (90%), especially sexual abuse, Herman (1992) suggested the term "complex post-traumatic stress disorder". The term clearly places high importance on trauma and gets away from the notion of personality disorder. The "complex" part refers to the fact that whilst a history of trauma is very significant and whilst there are similarities with

PTSD, there are also large differences. Clients who have a history of abuse have generally preferred this description, experiencing it as validating the importance and profound impact that trauma has had on their lives. Also a message is being received that "many people who went through what I did would have ended up this way". However, a problem with the term, is that 10% of clients who meet criteria for borderline personality disorder do not report a specific trauma history. A behavioural description of "emotion regulation disorder" is being explored as another alternative.

History of treatment

History of treatment had psychoanalysts finding a poor response to treatments available at the time. They concluded that treatment was not possible and stopped engaging these clients in treatment. Cognitive-behaviourists were focusing their treatment on clients who had well-defined target problems and who were more cooperative with treatment suggestions. There was little interest in the treatment of people meeting diagnostic criteria for borderline personality disorder. After a number of decades both groups modified their practices and began to successfully treat people meeting diagnostic criteria for borderline personality disorder with the area becoming increasingly a focus of research and treatment (see "Outcome studies" section). The belief that these clients were untreatable, whilst understandable at the time, has had far-reaching and long-lasting effects. It has been used to support individual and institutional policies of not providing resources and treatment; policies no longer tenable.

Epidemiology

Around 2% of the population are estimated to meet diagnostic criteria for borderline personality disorder. Swartz, Blazer, George and Winfield's (1990) study in North America found 1.8% of those aged 19–55 met criteria for borderline personality disorder. It could be estimated that around 0.5% of those meeting diagnostic criteria (or one in 10,000 people) will experience the severest difficulties. These are the people who are well known to public mental health services because of their frequent attendance at multiple treatment settings and who present public services with a challenge. Epidemiological studies in countries with significantly different cultures have yet to be carried out. Such studies could provide important information about aetiology. For example, would cultures with stronger affiliative connections with extended family and community as opposed to a nuclear family focus, have different prevalence rates?

There are people who believe we could be on the verge of an epidemic (Millon 1992; Millon 2000; Paris 1992; Paris 1996). This view is supported by evidence of an increase in suicide, youth suicide and people meeting criteria for diagnoses of antisocial personality disorder and substance use disorder, all of which are correlated with borderline personality disorder (Paris 1992). Nuclear families do not provide the same protection as extended family, from unskilled parenting and environmental influences. Paris (1992) writes,

> The hypothesis offered here is that social factors interact with other risk factors and promote BPD by lowering thresholds of impulsive behaviours. In an integrated social environment, social structures, which contain and modulate dysphoria, would act as a buffer to inner distress created by factors such as biological vulnerability, traumatic experiences and a dysfunctional family.

It is also quite likely that severity is increasing. The same socio-cultural reasons could be implicated. Also, many public mental heath services have admission for treatment criteria that ignore less severe behaviour and reinforce more severe behaviour. Clients know that in order to get treatment it is no longer sufficient to bruise yourself with your fists or cut your wrists as it has been in the past. Now you have to go to extremes. It is a challenge for policy planners to develop services with limited budgets that do not inadvertently create these problems.

The following is a summary of some current epidemiological data:

- ◆ 1.8% of the population meet criteria at any one point in time (Swartz *et al.*, 1990)
- ◆ People meeting criteria are well represented in mental health facilities, with estimates of 11% at community clinics and 20% in inpatient units (Swartz *et al.* 1990)

- 75% of those diagnosed are female (Swartz *et al.* 1990; Widiger and Frances 1989; Zanarini, Williams, Lewis *et al.* 1997; Zanarini, Frankenberg, Reich *et al.* 1999)
- Many authors believe males are under-represented and under-diagnosed in mental health settings and more likely to be found (but not diagnosed) in substance use centres and in the justice system
- 70% of those diagnosed have a history of sexual abuse (Herman, Perry and van der Kolk 1989; Ogata, Silk, Goodrich *et al.* 1990; Wideger and Francis 1989)
- 75% have a history of having self-harmed on at least one occasion (Dubo, Zanarini, Lewis, Williams 1997)
- 46% have a history being victims of adult violence (31% – rape, 33% – physical abusive partner) (Zanarini *et al.* 1999)
- There is considerable comorbidity (see "Comorbidity" section)

Diagnosis

Provided they are integrated with an individual understanding of the client, diagnosis and broad conceptualizations of borderline personality disorder can assist understanding and treatment. Two pragmatic conceptualizations of borderline personality disorder are provided followed by the formal DSM-IV criteria on which clinical diagnosis is typically established.

Beck, Freeman and associates (1990, pp. 186–187) name three core cognitive schema which have been shown to be stable over time (Arntz, Dietzel and Dreessen 1999): "The world is dangerous and malevolent", "I am powerless and vulnerable" and "I am inherently unacceptable" and describe how these schema interface,

> Some persons who view the world as a dangerous, malevolent place believe that they can rely on their own strengths and abilities in dealing with the threats it presents. However, borderline individuals' belief that they are weak and powerless blocks this solution. Other individuals who believe that they are not capable of dealing effectively with the demands of daily life resolve their dilemma by becoming dependent on someone who they see as capable of taking care of them (and develop a dependent pattern). However, borderlines' belief that they are inherently unacceptable blocks this solution, since this belief

leads them to conclude that dependence entails a serious risk of rejection, abandonment, or attack if this inherent unacceptability is discovered. Borderline individuals face quite a dilemma: convinced that they are relatively helpless in a hostile world but without a source of security, they are forced to vacillate between autonomy and dependence without being able to rely on either.

(Reprinted with the permission of Guilford Press.)

American psychologist Linehan (1993a), who developed DBT, describes clients as having high sensitivity to emotional stimuli (quick response at low thresholds), high reactivity (response is very large) and slow return to baseline (lengthy emotional arousal from previous stimulus contributes to high sensitivity). The metaphor of extensive burns to the skin comes to mind.

DSM-IV classifies personality disorder into Cluster A, B and C. Cluster A ("odd and eccentric") includes schizoid, schizotypal and paranoid personality disorder. Cluster B ("dramatic, emotional or erratic") includes histrionic, narcissistic, borderline and antisocial personality disorder. Cluster C ("anxious and fearful") includes avoidant, dependent and obsessive-compulsive personality disorder (American Psychiatric Association 1994).

People meeting criteria for a diagnosis in the Cluster C group are generally less impaired than those meeting criteria for a diagnosis in the Cluster B group and generally respond well to the usual psychotherapies. They are not generally the group of most concern to public mental health providers. People meeting criteria for a dominant diagnosis in the Cluster A group can have significant impairment but relatively infrequently seek out mental health services. People meeting criteria for a diagnosis in the Cluster B group are generally significantly impaired and of considerable concern to mental health providers.

Whilst questions remain about the validity of the diagnosis of borderline personality disorder, the behaviours described in DSM-IV criteria are well recognized by clinicians. Borderline personality disorder, as defined, is a multi-dimensional disorder which might be best considered as "severe personality dysfunction rather than a discrete entity" (Berelowitz and Tarnopolsky 1993) and with varying degrees of severity. A considerable percentage of the population have

Diagnostic criteria for borderline personality disorder – DSM-IV

(Reprinted with permission from the Diagnostic and Statistical Manual of Mental Disorders, Fourth Edition. Copyright 1994 American Psychiatric Association)

A pervasive pattern of instability of interpersonal relationships, self image, and affects, and marked impulsivity beginning by early adulthood and present in a variety of contexts, as indicated by five (or more) of the following:

1. frantic efforts to avoid real or imagined abandonment. Note: Do not include suicidal or self-mutilating behavior covered in Criterion 5
2. a pattern of unstable and intense interpersonal relationships characterised by alternating between extremes of idealization and devaluation
3. identity disturbance: markedly and persistently unstable self-image or sense of self
4. impulsivity in at least two areas that are potentially self damaging (e.g., spending, sex, substance abuse, reckless driving, binge eating). Note: Do not include suicidal or selfmutilating behavior covered in Criterion 5
5. recurrent suicidal behavior, gestures or threats or self mutilating behavior
6. affective instability due to a marked reactivity of mood (e.g., intense episodic dysphoria, irritability or anxiety usually lasting a few hours and only rarely more than a few days)
7. chronic feelings of emptiness
8. inappropriate intense anger or difficulty controlling anger (e.g., frequent displays of temper, constant anger, recurrent physical fights)
9. transient, stress related paranoid ideation or severe dissociative symptoms (American Psychiatric Association, 1994)

some traits. Having some so-called borderline personality disorder traits is probably a normal feature of adolescence. When the traits are of sufficient severity, a DSM-IV diagnosis can be made.

Persistently unstable or chaotic life-circumstances, impulsivity and affective instability may alert to the possibility of the diagnosis. To aid conceptualization, the DSM criteria can be grouped into three clusters:

Identity Cluster – feelings of emptiness, abandonment fears, unstable self-image or sense of self

Affective Cluster – inappropriate intense anger, affective instability, unstable and intense relationships

Impulse Cluster – self-harm, other impulsive behaviours (Hurt, Clarkin, Munroe-Blum and Marziali 1992)

Severe dissociation (Zanarini, Ruser, Frankenburg and Hennen 2000) and persistent self-harm are well correlated with a diagnosis of borderline personality disorder and are probably the two most discriminating features in making a diagnosis. Gunderson and Zanarini (1987) state that self-harm comes closest to being the "behavioral specialty" of people meeting diagnostic criteria for borderline personality disorder. Seventy-five percent of people meeting diagnostic criteria for borderline personality disorder have a history of at least one episode of self-harm (Dubo et al. 1997). Of course, neither self-harm nor severe dissociation is sufficient for the diagnosis. Many people self-harm or severely dissociate who do not have borderline personality disorder. The literature is less clear about what percentage of people who engage in an episode of self-harm meet diagnostic criteria for borderline personality disorder, as most studies of suicidal behaviour have not reported on Axis II diagnoses (Linehan 1993a).

Comorbidity

The high comorbidity with Axis I and II diagnoses and the unclear relationship with affective disorders lead to legitimate concerns about the validity of the diagnosis. Whilst these concerns are important and worthy of further research, it is critical that they do not distract from the need to treat people living with considerable morbidity.

Borderline personality disorder is probably best understood as a collection of symptoms and behaviours, that are present in a range of diagnoses and with considerable Axis I and Axis II comorbidity as highlighted below.

- Stone's (1989) study of people meeting diagnostic criteria for borderline personality disorder found only 37% had a "pure" diagnosis of borderline personality disorder (i.e. no comorbid diagnosis).

- There is considerable overlap between borderline personality disorder and affective disorders. The relationship remains one vigorously debated but not resolved (Swartz *et al.* 1990).

- A concurrent diagnosis of major depression was found in 71% of clients by Linehan (1993a), 70% by Bateman and Fonagy (1999) and 41% in a non-clinical sample by Swartz *et al.* (1990).

- A concurrent diagnosis of dysthymia was found in 63% of clients by Bateman and Fonagy (1999) and 24% by Linehan (1993a).

- A concurrent diagnosis of panic disorder was found in 50% of clients by Bateman and Fonagy (1999) and in 13% of a non-clinical sample by Swartz (1990).

- A concurrent diagnosis of agoraphobia was found in 36% of clients by Bateman and Fonagy (1999) and in 37% of a non-clinical sample by Swartz (1990).

- A concurrent diagnosis of bulimia was found in 38% of clients by Bateman and Fonagy (1999).

- Of those with a diagnosis of bulimia, 20–40% have been reported to meet criteria for borderline personality disorder, depending on sampling and diagnostic methods (Ames-Frankel, Devlin, Walsh *et al.* 1992).

- A high percentage of those attending drug and alcohol services meet criteria (Grilo, Martino, Walker *et al.* 1997; Dulit, Fyer, Haas *et al.* 1990). Reported prevalence rates of borderline personality disorder in substance users vary enormously depending on sampling factors, settings, diagnostic and assessment methods, time-frame and time of measurement (Trull, Sher, Minks-Brown *et al.* 2000; Verhuel, Hartgers, van den Brink and Koeter 1998). In a non-clinical sample, Swartz *et al.* (1990) found that of those people meeting diagnostic criteria for borderline personality disorder, 22% had a diagnosis of alcohol abuse and dependence and 50% had a lifetime history of drug problems.

◆ A majority of people meeting diagnostic criteria for borderline personality disorder also meet diagnostic criteria for another personality disorder (paranoid personality disorder – 30%, dependent personality disorder – 51%, avoidant personality disorder – 43%, antisocial personality disorder – 23%, histrionic personality disorder – 15%, narcissistic personality disorder – 16%) (Zanarini, Frankenberg, Dubo *et al.* 1998).

◆ There are suggestions of an overlap with a variety of organic brain disorders (Swartz *et al.* 1990).

Clinical boundaries

The histrionic, narcissistic and borderline diagnoses have a lot in common, with the borderline diagnosis being the most frequently made. The histrionic and narcissistic diagnoses are used much less now, in part because of pejorative, derogatory and, in the case of histrionic personality disorder, sexist associations. A person meeting diagnostic criteria for narcissistic personality disorder is generally more functional, less fragmented and more likely to be accessing private mental health services.

There is considerable overlap between borderline personality disorder and antisocial personality disorder. A pervasive failure of empathy is not a criteria in the DSM-IV diagnosis of antisocial personality disorder, but it was a clinically meaningful part of the old diagnostic terminology of psychopathy. People meeting diagnostic criteria for borderline personality disorder frequently have significant antisocial traits, but are able to be empathic to another's experience, sometimes exquisitely so, at least for short periods. People meeting diagnostic criteria for borderline personality disorder clearly have empathic capacity, often to a considerable degree, though it is not usually sustained and consistent and may occur only when things are going well.

People who are currently abusing drugs (especially illegal drugs) frequently have features of borderline personality disorder due to chaos, in many areas of their lives, related directly to substance use. This chaos can settle when substance use ceases. In these circumstances, a diagnosis needs to be made cautiously, preferably after drug use has stopped or the person, is for example, stabilized on methadone.

There is overlap between the symptoms of borderline personality disorder and bipolar affective disorder (Barbato and Hafner 1998; O'Connell, Mayo and Sciutto 1991; Pica, Edwards, Jackson *et al.* 1990). When the differential diagnosis includes borderline personality disorder and bipolar affective disorder, accurate diagnosis where possible will greatly improve outcome. An incorrect diagnosis of bipolar affective disorder encourages the clinician to overuse medication and to take too much responsibility. Once an inaccurate treatment culture has evolved, and staff, client and family expectations have developed, shifting diagnosis and treatment can be a very difficult process. The presenting symptoms of borderline personality disorder can be remarkably similar to those of a brittle, rapidly fluctuating form of bipolar disorder. People meeting diagnostic criteria for borderline personality disorder have affective shifts which tend to be of shorter duration, of more rapid onset and termination and more immediately linked to an identifiable environmental stressor with a strong interpersonal context.

The interface between psychotic phenomena and borderline personality disorder has generated considerable debate especially around implications for aetiology and classificatory systems, however the area remains unresolved. The presence of psychotic symptoms, whilst inviting consideration of an Axis I diagnosis of schizophrenia, is not sufficient for the diagnosis. Transient paranoid ideation is one of the DSM-IV diagnostic criteria for borderline personality disorder. The presence of hallucinations, pseudo hallucinations and brief psychotic episodes is not unusual in people meeting diagnostic criteria for borderline personality disorder without them meeting any of the other diagnostic criteria for schizophrenia. Research in the area has been limited with different definitions of psychotic phenomena. However there appears to be a higher than expected correlation between psychotic phenomena and PTSD (Butler, Mueser, Sorock and Braff 1996; Hamner, Frueh, Ulmer and Arana 1999; Ivezic, Oruc and Bell 1999; Sauter, Brailey, Uddo *et al.* 1999). There are suggestions of a similarly higher correlation between psychotic phenomena and borderline personality disorder (Dowson, Sussoms, Grounds and Taylor 2000; Miller, Abrams, Dulit and Fryer 1993).

There are dangers in making an incorrect Axis I or Axis II diagnosis. An incorrect diagnosis of borderline personality disorder may deprive the client of pharmacological treatment that is rapidly effective and relatively easy to institute for an Axis I disorder. Giving the client the "benefit of the doubt" and making a diagnosis of an Axis I disorder, till proven otherwise, may not always be in the interest of the client, as it might invite a client conceptualization that they are not responsible for their behaviour. A positive diagnosis of borderline personality disorder is ideally made without it being a diagnosis of exclusion, or a failure to respond to medications.

Aetiology

There are a number of factors correlated with borderline personality disorder. Zanarini *et al.* (1997) document 59% of clients retrospectively reporting childhood physical abuse, 92% childhood neglect and 29% prolonged childhood separation. Retrospective histories of sexual abuse are reported by about 70% of clients (Herman, Perry and van der Kolk 1989; Laporte and Guttman 1996; Ogata *et al.* 1990; Wideger and Francis 1989; Zanarini *et al.* 1997). Whilst sexual abuse is correlated with a diagnosis of borderline personality disorder, it is neither necessary (30% have no abuse history) nor sufficient (the vast majority of people who are sexually abused do not develop borderline personality disorder).

Neurophysiology of people meeting diagnostic criteria for borderline personality disorder is characterized by reduced serotonin activity (Coccaro 1998a; Woo-Ming and Siever 1998). Reduced serotonin activity has been linked with impulsivity, irritability, anger, lowered mood and suicide (Coccaro 1998a; Siever 1997; Silk 1997; Soloff 1997). It is possible that people who meet diagnostic criteria have a dysregulation of the noradrenergic system to stress, which could be linked with increased arousal, vigilance, anxiety, irritability and anger. Some studies (other studies have not been supportive) have found an increased incidence of brain trauma, childhood attention deficit hyperactivity disorder, neuro-cognitive impairment and learning disability (Gardner, Lucas and Cowdrey 1987; Lincoln, Bloom, Katz and Boxenbaum 1998; Van Reekum 1993; Van Reekum, Links, Finlayson et al. 1996; O'Leary 2000). There are strong suggestions of correlations with tempera-ment characterized by high emotional pain, impulsivity and limited affect regulation (Cloninger 1998). It is proposed that genetics significantly influences personality and that environmental factors (such as trauma) also impacts on neurophysiology (Cloninger 1998; Oldham 1997; Paris 1997; Paris 1998; Siever 1997; Zanarini and Frankenberg 1997). It has not been clearly shown, at this stage, how much the neurophysiological features are related to inborn physiology and how much a consequence of emotional trauma. Four articles in *Psychiatric Clinics of North America* (Gurvits, Koenigsberg and Siever 2000; O'Leary 2000; Oquendo and Mann 2000; Torgerson 2000) provide recent summaries on genetics, neurotransmitter function and neuropsychological testing in people with borderline personality disorder and an article on the biology of impulsivity, suicidality and self-harm.

Increasingly, researchers and theorists are proposing a complex multifactorial aetiological model embracing interacting predispos-ing and resilience factors with individuals having different pathways to developing the disorder (Figuero and Silk 1997; Paris 1998; Sabo 1997; Zanarini and Frankenberg 1997; Zanarini et al. 1997; Zanarini 2000). All theoretical schools have agreed about the aetiological importance of childhood abuse, neglect and invalidation. All schools are mindful of the neurophysiological factors but are in disagreement about the relative aetiological importance of these. It is plausible that people with a high genetic predisposition might require less environmental trauma to meet diagnostic criteria and people with severe repetitive environmental trauma might meet criteria with little or no genetic predisposition. It is likely that there are synergistic effects between genetic and environmental factors (Oldham 1997).

A hypothesis, which might apply to a number of clients, has a starting point of constitutionally vulnerable physiology to which is added childhood trauma. As a consequence of the trauma, relationships are affected and physiology and possibly brain "hard wiring" alters, decreasing learning capacity and increasing impulsivity, affective instability and hypersensitivity to stress. This, in turn, impacts on relationships. High sensitivity and reactivity to emotional stimuli, affective instability, fragmented identity development, poor object constancy, poor self-image, and dysfunctional schemas result and in time the behaviours and internal experiences of someone meeting diagnostic criteria for borderline personality disorder develop.

There are a number of hypotheses as to why females predominate: the incidence of sexual abuse; girls and women living in a marginalized, invalidating environment; the diagnosis being gender biased (the diagnosis is based on emotional expressivity which is higher amongst females); males with the same behaviours being more likely to receive a diagnosis of antisocial personality disorder; males with the same aetiological factors being more likely to be found in substance use services and to externalize their anger and end up in the justice system. There are strong suggestions that a significant percentage of perpetrators of domestic violence (who are more frequently male) would meet diagnostic criteria for borderline personality disorder, if assessed.

The diagram (Fig. 1.1) provides a visual summary of the points discussed.

Prognosis

Knowledge of prognosis has an important role in guiding treatment. Such knowledge can be of great assistance when clinicians doubt themselves, the appropriateness of the work they are doing and when challenged by colleagues about the appropriateness of the work. There have been people who have found this to be the single most useful piece of knowledge in the workshop on which this book is based, enabling them to retain hope when all appeared clinically dismal.

There are no absolutely naturalistic studies where people meeting diagnostic criteria for borderline personality disorder have been

Aetiology : Hypotheses

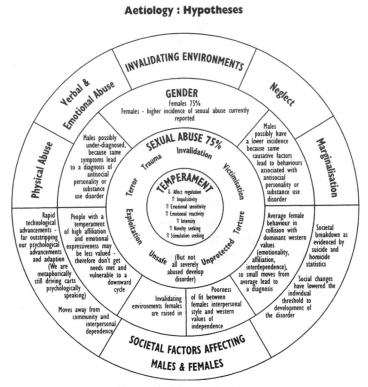

Fig. 1.1 Aetiology: hypotheses.

followed up without being treated, nor are there ever likely to be. The studies by Stone (1989), McGlashan (1986), Plakun, Burkhardt and Muller (1985) and Paris, Brown and Nowlis (1987) are considered to be as "naturalistic" as is possible. Being retrospective, these four studies are methodologically flawed, but have the credibility of obtaining similar results. Clients were followed up for 15 years or more. Level of function five years after discharge was poor and similar to people diagnosed with schizophrenia. Seventy-four percent of those who committed suicide had done so in the first five years after discharge (Stone, Stone and Hurt 1987; Stone 1990a; Stone 1993). After 15 years however, provided the clients had not committed suicide, people were doing reasonably well with two-thirds functioning "well" (GAS above 60), with most working and having a social life, whereas people with schizophrenia continued to function poorly (Stone 1989). Forty percent were considered cured (GAS above 70) (Stone, Stone and Hurt 1987; Stone 1989; Stone 1990a). Hospitalization had generally ceased after the first five years. Paris's study has now been extended from 15 to 27 years with further client improvements and only 8% still meeting criteria for borderline personality disorder (Paris and Zweig-Frank 2001).

In another study, Sabo, Gunderson, Najavits, Chauncey *et al.* (1985) prospectively monitored clients after a short inpatient treatment followed by outpatient individual psychotherapy carried out by whomever the client engaged. This study took place in a usual treatment as opposed to a rigorous research context and treatment was not monitored or standardised. At four-year follow–up, suicidal behaviour had decreased from 50% to 6%, however over 50% of participants were lost to follow-up.

Factors associated with a poorer prognosis are alcohol and substance use, comorbid major affective disorder, severity, antisocial traits or antisocial personality disorder, aggressivity and an absence of protective factors such as talent, attractiveness, high intelligence or self-discipline (Stone 1989; Stone 1990a). The presence of personality disorder also has an adverse impact on treatment outcomes for people with Axis I disorders (Reich and Vasile 1993).

The take-home message from the research is consistent with anecdotal information that people generally get better with time provided they don't kill themselves (obviously a big proviso). So, at a very minimum, if we are able to assist people with severe problems to stay alive, then we are probably being successful in our treatment. This mind shift from a string of short-term therapeutic failures to a successful long-term endeavour will counter the demoralization that often exists because the client is not "cured". A positive attitude is more likely to impact positively on client outcome. Linehan, (1995) speaking to a client, says,

> I'm telling you something, listen to me. If you don't kill yourself you are going to make it, you're going to get out of hell. You're going to get out of here; it's not always going to be so bad. Life is not always going to be so painful, and you're not going to hurt so bad. You're going to get to be a more normal person who has a life that's worth living. That's going to happen to you if you don't kill yourself. You

worked too hard, and you're too capable not to get there. You're going to get out; you just have to keep yourself alive.

(Reprinted with the permission of Guilford Press)

This perspective might also guide treatment planning and give support for long-term, intermittent treatment as an option if more continuous treatment is not possible because of client characteristics or resource considerations (see section "Duration of treatment").

Morbidity and mortality

The best way I have heard borderline personality disorder described is having been born without a skin - with no barrier to ward off real or perceived emotional assaults. What might have been a trivial slight to others was for me an emotional catastrophe.

(Williams 1998)

Morbidity

The high frequency of self-harm, substance abuse, anxiety disorders, depressive disorders and suicide are markers of the high morbidity that exists (see "Comorbidity" section). Clients' histories indicate a marked vulnerability to adult abuse, with 46% becoming victims of violence (rape – 31%; physically abusive partner – 33%) (Zanarini *et al.* 1999). Possible reasons for this include impulsivity, substance use, and limited capacity for self-protection (Zanarini *et al.* 1999). Koons *et al.*'s (2001) small study of women war veterans meeting diagnostic criteria for borderline personality disorder reported an even higher rate of adult abuse with 65% reported being battered by a partner and 85% being raped.

Mortality

The key findings on suicide are:

- ◆ The suicide rate of those presenting for treatment is 10% (Stone 1989; Plakun, Burkhardt and Muller 1985; Paris, Brown and Nowlis 1987; Kjelsberg, Eikeseth and Dahl 1991)
- ◆ This high mortality rate is similar to people meeting diagnostic criteria for schizophrenia or bipolar affective disorder (Stone 1989; Stone 1993)

♦ The rate rises to 36% with more severe forms of the disorder (8 out of 8 DSM-III criteria) (Stone 1989)

The suicide rate with the severest forms of the disorder might be higher still.

The above suicide rates were from an era before the publication of newer effective treatments (see "Outcome studies" section). These publications have client numbers too small to comment on the treatment's impact on suicide, however it is a reasonable hypothesis that these approaches are associated with lower suicide rates.

As the majority who suicide will do so in the first five years after presentation, it is likely that the rate of suicide in this period is higher for those with a borderline personality disorder diagnosis than any other mental health diagnosis. A Swedish study of 58 consecutive suicides among 15–29 year-olds, showed that one-third would have met diagnostic criteria for borderline personality disorder, which was the most common psychiatric diagnosis, higher than that of depression (Runeson and Beskow 1991; Runeson, Beskow and Waern 1996). A similar Canadian study of 75 consecutive suicides in 18–35 year old males found that 28% would have met criteria for borderline personality disorder (Lesage, Boyer, Grunberg *et al.* 1994).

Considerable recent attention has been placed on the early treatment of people meeting diagnostic criteria for schizophrenia. There is sufficient information indicating the appropriateness of similar attention being placed on early intervention in those presenting with borderline personality disorder. Linehan (1997) writes that, "12 to 33% of all individuals who die by suicide meet criteria for BPD". The suicide rate is only slightly "less than patients with depression, alcoholism or schizophrenia, making it one of the most lethal of psychiatric disorders" (Soloff 1997).

Health resource usage

Swartz *et al.* (1989) demonstrated higher use of mental health services than people from other mental health diagnostic groups, except for people meeting diagnostic criteria for schizophrenia, whose utilization rates were similar. Sansone, Sansone and

Wiederman (1996) demonstrated higher than average health care utilization in primary care settings. Morton and Buckingham (1994) documented inpatient and community health resource usage of 91 people meeting diagnostic criteria for borderline personality disorder, who made the most use of services in Victoria, Australia (population 4.5 million). Over a two-year period, the average cost of treatment for each of these 91 people was $A59,340 (1994/95 cost estimates) with approximately 90% of costs for inpatient care (1994). Similarly high hospitalization rates for the highest users of service were found by Krawitz (1997a) (139.2 days/client per year) and Perry (1996) (56.6 days/client per year). Clients in the Stevenson and Meares' (1992) study (see section "Psychosocial treatments") used a mean of 86.1 days in hospital in the year prior to treatment.

Clients are often receiving treatment in a reactive manner without a specific proactive treatment package and are already high users of services. The problem with current health resource usage is that much of it goes into crisis treatment, which fails to address the evidence that long-term treatment planning is required for effective outcomes.

Health resource use after effective treatment

In Linehan, Armstrong, Suarez and Allmon's (1991) study, the DBT group used 31 less hospital days/client than the control group. Stevenson and Meares' (1992) study demonstrated a reduction of 42 (86–44) hospital days/client in the year following treatment. A retrospective cost analysis of the Stevenson and Meares (1999) study showed a reduction of hospital costs of $A21,431/client in the year following treatment. The one year of treatment, with costs of the therapy factored in, resulted in a net health resource usage reduction of $A8,431/client. Bateman and Fonagy's (2001) study demonstrates less hospital use over a three year period in the experiment versus the control group (1.7 vs. 15.8 days), but overall cost-effectiveness was not reported on. A review of the economic impact of psychotherapy calculates DBT saving approximately $US10,000/patient/year (Gabbard, Lazar, Hornberger and Spiegel 1997). The review concludes that psychotherapy in the treatment of borderline personality disorder has a beneficial effect on costs, particularly through the decreased use of hospitalization, and, in Stevenson and Meares' study, increased time at work (Gabbard *et al.* 1997). In Stevenson and Meares' (1992) study there was a mean reduction of 93 days away from work (134−41) and a reduction of 36 medical visits (42−6) in the year following treatment. To change the pattern of resource usage away from hospitalization, significant resources need to be allocated for proactive community treatment.

Different treatment models

A variety of psychotherapy models have been used to treat this client group. Brief introductions to different psychotherapy models are provided below.

Psychodynamic and psychoanalytically informed psychotherapy

Psychodynamic theorists view the client as having a poorly formed or fragmented identity due to incomplete or disrupted psychological developmental in childhood. Normal development involves the early establishment of a secure attached relationship. From this solid base, the child can develop a sense of self whilst psychologically separating and individuating. Problems developing a secure attachment, or with separation and individuation, can lead to insecure ambivalent attachments and problems with development of identity and sense of self. If these problems progress into adulthood, there will be a poor sense of self, poorly formed identity and associated problems with self-esteem. Relationships may be associated with avoidance, intense ambivalence, or with loss of identity and individuality.

A stage of normal development is learning to integrate conflicting feelings such as like and dislike for the same person. If psychological development in this area is impeded, adult relationships may be associated with polarization (on–off; love you–hate you). The person may "split" themselves, so to speak, into different parts, with each part dominant at any one time and with limited capacity to integrate the constituent parts into a cohesive whole.

People are related to as part-people, rather than integrated whole people. People will be perceived of as either all-gratifying or all-persecuting with associated idealization and devaluation.

Treatment is based on these developmental understandings. The therapist's goal is to develop a relationship with the client that will serve to sustain the therapy, be the core focus of the therapy and be the primary agent of change. The therapy relationship is, accordingly, given priority in planning and provision of treatment. It is expected that the therapy relationship will be a source of considerable understanding for client and clinician. It is likely that the client will behave towards and have feelings for the therapist, which are repetitions of past important relationships (transference), which may include idealization and devaluation. Some of the behaviours and feelings in the client–therapist relationship may be constructive to achieving client goals and others counter-productive. The task, in many psychodynamic therapies, is to "bring to light of day", client behaviours and feelings for exploration in order to achieve client goals. The client increasingly becomes aware of an inner world that they can reflect on. Through the emotional exploration of these feelings, in the context of a safe therapy relationship, the client achieves better understanding and knowledge of themselves, associated with a more stable, secure sense of identity. This is linked with a more cohesive integration of internal parts and less idealization and devaluation. The client, also, can explore alternative more constructive ways of relating, thereby breaking past repetitive cycles.

The therapist, too, will have feelings towards the client. Some of these feelings may be constructive, others not so. Therapist feelings may inform about the client or may be more about the therapist. All these therapist feelings, in the broadest sense of the word, are countertransference. The therapist needs to reflect upon their feelings, during the session and in supervision, attempting to make use of their feelings to better understand and treat the client.

One of the major tasks of the psychodynamic therapist is to assist the client to feel metaphorically contained (not be overwhelmed by feelings) and "held". The therapist provides a "containing", "holding" function via a relationship that is consistent, continuous, solid and predictable and one that the client experiences as empathic and respectful. This "holding" function provides the foundation of a connected relationship out of which self-definition and identity develop.

Treatment and the therapy relationship progress along lines of psychological development. Early stages may centre around attachment, engagement and attempts to establish a secure relationship base. Part of this exploration will include issues of separation and individuation, which will carry on throughout much of the therapy. The goal of treatment is for the client to develop over a period of time, via the relationship with the therapist, the capacity to flexibly integrate intimacy and autonomy, self-worth, who they are (identity) and a clear sense of purpose.

Self psychology

Psychodynamic treatment models, and self psychology in particular, have evolved over the years to focus less on interpretation and more on empathy. The task is not merely for the therapist to be empathic, but for the client to feel that the therapist is empathic to their experience. The goal is for the client to feel that the therapist is alert and responsive to the client's moment-to-moment feelings, never giving up on trying to understand the client's reality and where necessary, putting this understanding into words. To achieve this, the therapist focuses on all information which will alert them to empathic attunement or its failure. Whilst the task of empathy is crucial, so too is the task of repair of empathic failures. Failures of attunement are inevitable and in many situations will be obvious, such as a client overtly and angrily criticizing the therapist. Many times however, the therapist has to be alert for subtle signs of misattunement. This may manifest in moment-to-moment changes in a client's voice (volume, tone, modulation), body posture, facial expression, eye contact, language and affect. The therapist needs to silently note these markers, reflect upon them and consider a response which will re-establish empathic attunement.

In self psychology especially, the relationship between client and clinician is viewed as an alive, constantly evolving interactional process significantly influenced by both client and therapist. This intersubjective space, more than the client or therapist alone, is the focus of therapeutic exploration as a single system. The therapist needs to create a safe and secure place where the client's inner world and self can begin to emerge. This occurs in an environment where the client is aware of the supportive unobtrusive presence of another person (Meares 1993; Meares 1996).

Relationship management

Relationship management developed by Dawson (1988, Dawson and MacMillan 1993) emphasizes the interactional nature of client and clinician behaviours. Clinicians are encouraged to be aware of process (as opposed to content) communications to the therapist, whereby the client attempts to define themself in the sick role ("incompetent, helpless, not responsible"). Undue response to these communications ("transactions") can reinforce this sick role whilst the therapist or treating team take on the complimentary role of having "control", "competence" and "responsibility" (Dawson 1988). A possible end point of such "transactions" is use of mental health legislation where the clinician overtly assumes responsibility for the client and the client's behaviour. The therapist, using a relationship management model, advises the client that the therapist will be a consistent, warm, active listener but is unsure of being able to be helpful beyond that ("No therapy therapy") (Dawson and MacMillan 1993). Dawson (1988) states that the therapists, by their actions, communicates to the client "that she is a healthy, competent, intelligent, responsible, likeable adult. Her behavior and then her sense of self will gradually adopt this definition".

Cognitive analytic therapy (CAT)

CAT is a model that has been developed in Britain and is an amalgam of object relations theory and cognitive models. The therapy focuses on the narrative the client brings to the therapy, out of which a re-formulation of the clients' experience is described. The description is documented in both narrative and diagrammatic form. The client and therapist keep the client file, and the therapy is goal focused with a homework component. Treatment is focused on the understanding and changing of patterns of behavior. Treatment explores the overview of the life of the client. Explanations are developed for the client's perpetuating patterns of unhelpful behavior, which are maintained because they were once useful. The exploration of the patterns operating in the relationship with the therapist and the investment in homework tasks provide the opportunities for change.

Psychoanalytic theorists

Kernberg (1975)	Believes problem is one of intrapsychic conflict with a core of aggressivity. Treatment tends to be challenging.
Masterson (1976)	Focus is more interpersonal with a challenging style to orientate client to reality.
Kohut (1977)	(Self psychology) Believes problem to be one of intrapsychic deficit. Treatment is softer and focuses on empathy, repair of inevitable empathic failures and positive affiliation.
Gunderson (1984)	Pragmatic individual psychodynamic therapy. In addition may integrate separate case management, skills training, medication and family psychoeducation (1999, 2001).
Adler (1985)	Believes problem is one of intrapsychic deficit.
Benjamin (1993)	Strong focus on the interpersonal area.
Meares (1993)	(Self psychology) Focus on empathic attunement. Special focus on creating a relaxed environment for client to experience their inner world and develop self.

Cognitive-behavioural therapies

Over the last 15 to 20 years there has been the development of some cognitive behavioural therapies. DBT is the most well known with a robust emerging research base and has been trialed with individuals with severe symptoms. There are however several other models emerging.

Dialectical behavior therapy (DBT)

DBT (Linehan 1993a) has behavioural therapy at its core with contributions from cognitive therapy, eastern psychological practices and paying considerable attention to the relationship between client and clinician. There is a continual attention to the engagement and commitment of the client to treatment and treatment goals. DBT views the client as having a core problem regulating affect. The core treatment involves behaviour chain analysis and skills training. Identified problem behaviours such as suicidality and self-harm are the focus of behavioural chain analyses followed by a solution analysis looking at more effective alternatives. Skills training is conducted in an education format with the clients being formally taught the skills. The skills training classes are structured and have appropriate teaching methods applied. For many clinicians there is no possibility of setting up a group but the skills can be taught to individuals. Skills training uses a mixture of self-acceptance skills and change skills as outlined in the box below.

DBT has been modified for work in inpatient, day programs, family, substance use, violence and eating disorders. As well as its demonstrated efficacy in treating people meeting diagnostic criteria for borderline personality disorder, there has been one trial of its efficacy with substance use (Linehan, Schmidt, Dimeff *et al.* 1999) and one trial of its efficacy in the treatment of bulimia (Safer, Telch and Agras 2001.

Dialectical behavior therapy (DBT)
(Linehan, 1993a)

Dialectics – the synthesis of opposites. The task is for client, clinician and organization to synthesise dichotomous, black/white, absolutist, all-or-nothing thinking. To move from "either/or" to "both and". The major dialectic in DBT is that clients "radically accept" themselves as they are and at the same time explore ways of changing themselves and their lives.

Individual therapy

1 hour/week
Therapy tasks include:

Negotiating and contracting about treatment
Motivational interviewing
Problem and solution analysis (see "Behaviour chain and solution analysis" section)

Group therapy (skills training)

$2\frac{1}{2}$ hours/week

Mindfulness skills (attention skills: observe, describe and then participate)
   Observing and describing decreases impulsivity, increases capacity for self-reflection and provides data for behavioural chain analysis. Observing without judgement can increase self-acceptance. Observing distress without acting can lead to the recognition that distress can be tolerated or even pass without direct action. Attention skills increase capacity to choose to distract, which is a highly effective means of regulating emotion

Distress tolerance skills – Distracting, self-soothing, improving the moment, thinking of pros and cons, "radical" acceptance of distress

Emotion regulation skills – Including myths about emotion and learning to identify emotions "observe and describe"

Dialectical behavior therapy (DBT)
(Linehan, 1993a) *(cont.)*

Interpersonal effectiveness skills – Assertiveness – Focus on saying "no" and asking for what you want

Telephone calls

Encouraged to make appropriate brief calls for the following reasons:

- Encourage overt communication rather than covert communication such as self-harm
- To get assistance or "coaching" in how to better use the skills learnt in therapy
- Assist generalising of skills into the real community of the client
- To assist repair of therapeutic alliance

Consultation meeting to the therapist

- Peer group supervision
- The same strategies used for the client are used for therapists

Ancillary treatments

e.g. hospitalization, day program, medication, self-help groups

Treatment priorities

1. Suicide and self-harm behaviours
2. Therapy interfering behaviours – on the part of the client or therapist (e.g. client – not turning up for appointments; clinician – resenting seeing the client)
3. Behaviours interfering with quality of life – especially those leading to crises (e.g. substance abuse, inability to make friends, staying in abusive relationships, not getting necessary medical care, disabling anxiety)
4. Posttraumatic stress therapy (exploration of past traumas)

Schema-focused therapy (Young 1997)

Schema-focused therapy is an integrative therapy with cognitive therapy at its core, with extensive influence from object relations and gestalt therapies.

Four dominant shifting dimensions of the client are identified, with each dimension having an associated structured treatment strategy.

1. The "abandoned child" dimension requires the therapist to empathize with the client and to assist the client to nurture themselves.
2. The "angry child" dimension requires therapist empathy balanced with appropriate limit-setting and reality testing. The therapist assists the client to find healthier ways of expressing anger.
3. The "punitive parent" dimension refers to that part of the client that is self-critical and requires the therapist to assist the client to fight off and get rid of the "punitive parent".
4. The "detached protector" refers to that part of the client that is emotionally detached to protect against excessive pain. The "detached protector" needs reassurance that it is OK to feel. This can be done by timely exploration of painful memories and by dealing with the "abandoned, angry and punitive child" dimensions.

Commonalities between different models

Different models tend to have firm, explicit contracts, a high degree of clinician engagement and a proactive, disciplined approach to impulsive behaviour (Allen 1997; Milton, Dawson, Kazmierczak et al. 1999). All models highlight the importance of the client–clinician relationship, of the therapeutic alliance and of patterns of client behaviours manifesting in the client–clinician relationship (Allen 1997; Milton et al. 1999). All models require clinicians to remain relatively calm in crisis, be mindful of their feelings and to set limits to assist the clinician in maintaining warmth for the client, so essential for a positive outcome (Allen 1997; Milton *et al.* 1999).

In exploring similarities in four different models, Allen (1997) notes the acceptance that therapists will make errors, which need to be acknowledged (perhaps with a brief apology) and used if possible to therapeutic advantage. A client (Jackson 1999) writes, "People make mistakes – admit them. I will probably know anyway and then you are denying my reality. I also like to know you are human". Allen (1997) notes that all four models encourage clinicians to interact in a manner that minimizes the client feeling criticized. At the same time, however, he also states "all four paradigms caution against treating the patient as if he or she were fragile or incapable of being reasonable...". It is important for clinicians to be well grounded in the theory and practice of the model they are using. There is a place for using an integrative model provided this, too, is well grounded and not an ad hoc, reactive approach.

Multimodel approach

A multimodel integrative approach draws flexibly and with careful consideration from different models to meet each individual client's needs. (This is very different from the notion of throwing something at the problem hoping that eventually there will be a positive effect). DBT integrates different core models and is based in behavioural and to a lesser degree cognitive theory and practice, whilst placing maximum importance on the therapy relationship. Young's schema–focused therapy also uses a multimodel approach, integrating cognitive behavioural, object relations and action therapy models. Gunderson (2001) describes the complimentary nature of having different models (case management, pharmacology, cognitive-behavioural and psychodynamic) available to best match treatment with the client's current level of function. In *"Treatment of borderline patients: a pragmatic approach"* Stone (1990b) writes,

> ...borderline patients have a way of reducing us to our final, common, human denominator, such that allegiance to a rigidly defined therapeutic system becomes difficult to maintain. They force a shift in us, as it were, from the dogmatic to the pragmatic (1990b).

He writes of the ABCDE of a multimodel approach: A – analytic, B – behavioural, C – cognitive, D – drug, E – eclectic (1990b).

An organizing clinical framework for mental health clinicians

Mental health clinicians have extensive skills to draw on. Positive outcomes can be achieved when these skills are integrated into a considered clinical plan based on principles of effective treatments. Of course, intensive training in the evidence-based treatments is desirable, but not necessary nor practical for all clinicians in a mental health service. The following tables are an outline of a clinical framework that is available to general mental health clinicians using existing workforce skills.

An organizing clinical framework for mental health clinicians

Case management

- ◆ Develop, carry out and review clinical plan (includes establishing goals, contracting and monitoring treatment)
- ◆ Coordinate treatment
- ◆ Clarify different clinicians' roles
- ◆ Communicate with all relevant parties

Crisis theory and practice

(adapted for the area of borderline personality disorder)

Skills acquisition

- ◆ Cognitive behaviour therapy skills
- ◆ Problem solving skills

Rehabilitation

- ◆ Social supports – people
- ◆ Social supports – money
- ◆ Social supports – accommodation
- ◆ Psychoeducation

An organizing clinical framework for mental health clinicians *(cont.)*

Supportive psychotherapy

- "Real" relationship between therapist and client
- Day-to-day realities – does not explore past as major part of treatment
- Practical
- Psychoeducation, skills training
- Advice, praise and encouragement where therapeutic

Milton and Banfai (1999 pp. 3–4) write that where clinicians are not trained in a specific model such as DBT or self psychology,

> ... a supportive psychotherapy is probably the easiest to maintain, allowing for a workable combination of different interventions within a coherent model of care. In this way of working, the clinician acts as a secure base, strengthening the client's adaptive functioning through suggestion, education, limit setting and facilitating therapeutic alliance. Creation of the alliance over the long term, coupled with consistency and availability, may be of greater importance to success with the client than any of the specific therapeutic interventions themselves.

Supportive psychotherapy

Aims

- Adaptation in the present
- Long-term change through improved day-to-day functioning

Goals/outcomes

- Realistic, practical/pragmatic, here and now
- Stabilization and then change
- Increased knowledge and understanding of strengths and weaknesses
- Maximize strengths, minimize weaknesses

Supportive psychotherapy *(cont.)*

Structure of treatment

- Frequency and regularity fluid and dependent on need
- Duration variable – may be short/long/intermittent/ indefinite
- Finishing – generally slow, attenuated, as long as necessary
- Reliability and availability of therapist – high

Theory

- Integration and synthesis from different models (especially psychodynamic, cognitive, behavioural, Rogerian)
- Therapist as explicit attachment figure
- Positive client–therapist relationship is crucial
- Change will flow from a positive therapeutic relationship
- Interpersonal principles

Values

- Common sense, practicality
- Can be OK to suppress/repress distressing material
- "Being there" with the client
- Believing in the client
- Celebrate joys, skills, successes, and strengths
- "Heroism of simply coping" (Holmes 1995)
- "Celebrating the ordinary" (Holmes 1995)
- People respond/change when treated with dignity, respect and support

Style

- Conversational
- Soothing
- Low intensity

Techniques

- Empathic, active listening, warmth, positive interest

Supportive psychotherapy (cont.)

- ◆ Skills training (especially self-soothing, mood modulation, problem solving)
- ◆ Cognitive behaviour therapy skills, psychoeducation
- ◆ Maximize adaptive strategies/behaviours (e.g. distraction)
- ◆ Minimize less adaptive strategies/behaviours (e.g. self-harm)
- ◆ Praise, encouragement, reassurance, suggestion and advice where appropriate
- ◆ Contingency planning (limit-setting)
- ◆ Dilute transference, rapid intervention in negative transference

Clinician

- ◆ Real (vs. therapist persona), active (vs. passive), transparent (vs. opaque)
- ◆ More self-disclosure
- ◆ Countertransference issues even more important because therapist more visible

Outcome studies

Psychosocial treatments

The evidence-based research review organization, the Cochrane Collaboration has not done a systematic review on borderline personality. There is a growing literature base on evidenced-based outcome studies. In 1998 in *"A guide to treatments that work"*, a text focused on evidence-based research, Crits-Christoff (1998) named only two randomized controlled trials published at the time. By the end of 2001 there have been a further four randomized controlled trials published making six randomized controlled trials published to date (Linehan *et al.* 1991; Linehan, Schmidt, Dimeff *et al.* 1999; Munroe-Blum and Marziali 1995; Bateman and Fonagy 1999; Turner 2000; Koons, Robins, Tweed *et al.* 2001). In addition there is one waiting list controlled study published (Stevenson and Meares 1992; Stevenson and Meares 1999). These studies are described below in order of date of publication.

Linehan *et al.*'s (1991; Linehan, Heard and Armstrong 1993c) randomized, controlled trial demonstrated significant improvements in the DBT versus treatment as usual group on measures of self-harm, hospitalization, social adjustment, anger and general functioning after one year of treatment. The DBT group had a 60% reduction of self-harm and a reduction of hospital days of 39 days (control-8 days) in the one year of treatment. In DBT, the client is enouraged to use brief telephone calls to the individual therapist at behaviourally relevant times (e.g. before self harming). There was a low use of telephone calls in both groups with a moderate but non-statistically significant higher use for the DBT group (2.4 calls/client/month) compared to the control group (1.6 calls/client/month) (Linehan and Heard 1993d).

Stevenson and Meares (1992), in a prospective study, treated clients twice weekly for one year using a self psychology model. Results demonstrated a decrease in violent behaviour by 70%, medical visits by 87%, self-harm episodes by 78%, hospital admissions by 59%, hospital days by 49% (86.1 days−44.1 days) and there was a significant reduction in symptoms measured on a self-administered rating scale. Treated clients made significant gains on a score derived from DSM criteria whereas the control group (treatment as usual while on waiting list) were unchanged (Meares, Stevenson and Comerford 1999).

Munroe-Blum and Marziali (1995), in a randomized control trial, treated clients for 30 ninety-minute sessions using a modified form of psychodynamic group psychotherapy (interpersonal group psychotherapy based on Dawson's relationship management model) versus twice-weekly individual psychodynamic psychotherapy. Both groups made equally significant improvements measured on self-administered rating scales, but the experiment group treatment was cheaper. It appears the study population had less severe difficulties than the clients in the Linehan and Stevenson/Meares studies with only one-third having a history of suicide attempt (not defined) and one-third with a history of hospitalization.

Bateman and Fonagy's (1999) randomized controlled trial of clients treated with 18 months partial hospitalization (day program) demonstrated greater improvements than standard psychiatric care (case management without psychotherapy) on a range of measures, with most changes beginning after 6 months of treatment. The experimental group had a decreased number of self-harm episodes (9 fold decrease in median number of episodes) and clients attempting suicide (95% pre-treatment and 5% post-treatment in previous 6 months). Anxiety, depression and social adjustment were significantly better in the experimental group. Clients were treated with a psychoanalytically orientated intervention which integrated individual and group therapy provided by psychiatric nurses who had no formal psychotherapy qualifications. Partial hospitalization was used to balance support and individual responsibility aiming to be "neither too much nor too little" (Bateman and Fonagy 1999). The experimental group showed a statistically significant continued improvement in the 18 months post partial hospitalization when they received two hours/week group psychotherapy. During the 3 years of treatment reported, the experimental group used less full hospitalization (mean 1.7 days/client vs. 15.6 days/client) (Bateman and Fonagy 2001).

A randomized controlled trial of DBT versus treatment as usual for people meeting diagnostic criteria for borderline personality disorder and drug dependence demonstrated significantly greater reduction in drug use after one year of treatment and at 16-month follow-up in the DBT compared to the treatment as usual group. The DBT group maintained subjects better in treatment and had significantly greater gains in global and social adjustment (Linehan, Schmidt, Dimeff et al. 1999).

A randomized controlled trial of one year of DBT-oriented therapy versus client centred therapy demonstrated significantly greater improvements on suicidal thinking, self-harm behaviours, impulsivity, anger, depression, global functioning and days in hospital in the DBT group (Turner 2000). The modifications to DBT were the inclusion of a psychodynamic formulation and DBT skills training being provided by the individual therapist (not in a group as in the original 1991 study by Linehan et al.). Of interest was the finding that the quality of the therapeutic alliance accounted for as much variance in improvement as the differences in the treatment conditions.

A randomized controlled trial of DBT versus treatment as usual was conducted over six months of treatment (Koons, Robins, Tweed *et al.* 2001). Those in DBT reported significantly greater decreases in suicidal ideation, hopelessness, depression and anger expression. Only the DBT group demonstrated significant decreases in self-harm, anger experienced but not expressed and dissociation and a strong trend on the number of hospitalizations. This study represents the first published DBT replication study done outside of the originators of DBT (Linehan in Seattle).

Other studies are methodologically weaker, or the client group studied included people meeting diagnostic criteria for personality disorders other than borderline personality disorder. Barley, Buie, Peterson *et al.* (1993) demonstrated a three-fold decrease in self-harm episodes, using a DBT model in a part-prospective, part-retrospective controlled study of an inpatient unit (median length of stay – 106 days). In another study, preliminary pre–post data after one year of DBT treatment showed decreases of hospital days by 77%, face to-face contact with emergency services by 80% and treatment costs by 58% (American Psychiatric Association 1998). A three month hospitalization using DBT prior to out patient DBT treatment in an uncontrolled pilot study showed significant improvements on a number of ratings including parasuicidal acts (Bohus, Haaf, Stiglmayr *et al.* 2000). A preliminary report by Chiesa and Fonagy (2000) on their ongoing study of psychosocial treatment at the Cassel, compared the outcomes of clients treated with six months residential treatment followed by community outreach and group psychotherapy with a non-randomized controlled group receiving residential treatment (11–16 months) only. Both groups improved, with the experimental group showing statistically larger improvements on two measures (Global Assessment Scale, Social Adjustment Scale). Ryle and Golynkina report on outcomes of clients treated in a naturalistic uncontrolled trial with 24 sessions (plus 4 follow-up sessions) of cognitive analytic therapy. Significant improvements on the Beck Depression Inventory and Symptom Checklist 90-R are reported post-treatment and at 18-month post-treatment (Ryle and Golynkina 2000). These results after a relatively brief treatment are encouraging not only in terms of efficacy but also efficiency. A pilot study of positive outcomes with a series of five patients treated with cognitive analytic therapy has also been reported (Wildgoose, Clarke and Waller 2001). An uncontrolled one-year trial of Kernberg's modified psychodynamic treatment (called transference-focused psychotherapy) showed a significant decrease in the number of clients attempting suicide and fewer hospitalizations. Whilst there was not a significant difference in the number of self-injurious behaviours, there was a significant difference in the severity of medical risk following self-injury. Seventy-four percent were retained in treatment (Clarkin, Foelsch, Levy *et al.* 2001).

There are four positive prospective outcome studies where clients were used as their own controls, which took place in residential, semi-residential or day programs. Tucker, Bauer, Wagner *et al.* (1987), Vaglum, Friis, Irion *et al.* (1990) and Hafner and Holme's (1996) treatment were psychodynamic, all using therapeutic community principles. Krawitz's (1997b) study had only six clients with a borderline personality disorder diagnosis and used a treatment package that included psychodynamic, cognitive-behavioural, and sociopolitical approaches. Nehls (1994) reported on a trial of five clients who essentially were in charge of their brief acute hospital admission rights. Results showed a 47% decrease in the number of days in hospital (25.8–13.8/client for the year).

Other models showing promise but as yet without published data demonstrating efficacy are schema-focused therapy developed by Young (research in progress) and case management/rehabilitation/ supportive psychotherapy. Case management/rehabilitation/sup-portive psychotherapy draws strongly from and modifies case management and rehabilitation models used for people meeting diagnostic criteria for schizophrenia and bipolar affective disorder and makes use of supportive psychotherapy practices (Links 1993; Nehls and Diamond 1993). Strengths of this model are workforce availability and likely acceptability.

The Cochrane Collaboration (Hawton, Arensman, Townsend *et al.* 1998) completed a systematic review of treatments for deliberate self-harm. This review reports significantly reduced self-harm for two treatments: depot flupenthixol and DBT; and non-significant trends towards reduced self-harm for two treatments: problem-solving therapy and the provision of an emergency contact card. The review states, "The results of this systematic review indicate that currently there is insufficient evidence on which to make firm recommendations about the most effective forms of treatment for patients who have recently engaged in deliberate self-harm. This is a serious situation given the size of the problem of deliberate self-harm throughout the world and its importance for suicide prevention" (Hawton *et al.*, 1998).

In a pilot study, clients with a history of repeated deliberate self-harm who received brief cognitive therapy (containing elements of DBT) after an episode of self-harm had fewer suicidal acts, were less depressed and used 46% less healthcare resources over the following 6 months than the treatment as usual control group (Evans, Tyrer, Catalan *et al.* 1999). The brevity of the intervention (mean – 2.7 sessions) suggests its feasibility as a broad based public health measure. Salkovskis, Ather and Storer using a problem solving approach reported similar results with clients who had "repeated suicide attempts" in a randomized controlled trial (1990).

There is limited information to guide clinicians about different treatment models for people with different levels of severity of borderline personality disorder. DBT, Bateman/Fonagy's psycho-analytically orientated partial hospitalization and Stevenson/Meares' self psychology are the best researched treatment models for people meeting diagnostic criteria for severe forms of borderline personality disorder. The Linehan *et al.* (1991) study appears to have had a population with a considerably higher baseline rate of self-harm than the Stevenson/Meares (1992) study with the Bateman/Fonagy (1999) study having intermediate levels. The Linehan, Stevenson/Meares and Bateman/Fonagy studies demonstrated an important capacity to maintain clients in treatment with retention rates of 83–86%, well above the 50% figure previously considered acceptable. Gunderson (1999) suggests a treatment trajectory using DBT, case management and medication, singly or in combination, where clients are unable to control impulses and feelings. When the client is more stable, they will have an opportunity to move on to other psychotherapy treatments.

In summary, there are six randomized controlled trials published. DBT has the most research data with three randomized controlled trials and one randomized controlled trial of a modified form of DBT. All the researched treatments can guide current practices, which can evolve as new data becomes available. Current trials of DBT, psychodynamic psychotherapy, residential therapy, cognitive analytic therapy, case management/supportive psychotherapy are underway and will provide much-needed information over the next few years. The very limited treatment outcome studies (and only two published replications – DBT) is short of the desired standard. Nevertheless, there is an accumulating body of information that treatment can be effective. This research base will, almost certainly, be consolidated over the next few years. Not providing services till the data meets the standard we would like is overly cautious and will continue the perpetuating, self-reinforcing cycle of poor outcomes and negativity.

Pharmacological treatments

Like psychosocial treatments, the pharmacological treatment of people meeting diagnostic criteria for borderline personality disorder has advanced in the last 15 years but still remains in its infancy. Research is difficult because of the high comorbidity and the natural history of rapid fluctuations in symptoms. Trials are few, have shown only modest gains or cannot be replicated. This tends to confirm current anecdotal clinical experience, that pharmacological treatment, if used, should not dominate treatment but should serve as an adjunct to psychosocial treatments. The American Psychiatric Association (2001) guidelines describe and support the common clinical situation of psychosocial and pharmacological treatments being used in tandem. Of course, comorbid conditions such as major depressive episode need to be treated in their own right. The American Psychiatric Association (2001) guidelines provide a recent review of pharmacological treatment. Other reviews have been provided by Coccaro (1998a), Hirschfield (1997), Links, Heslegrave and Villella (1998), Soloff

(2000) and Woo-Ming and Siever (1998). Gabbard has written a chapter on combining medication with psychotherapy (2000). Together with Soloff's article (2000) this provides a complimentary and synthesized update from an expert in psychoanalytic psychotherapy (Gabbard) and from an expert in the biological treatment of borderline personality disorder (Soloff).

Serotonergic agents

Therapists perceived a decrease in client impulsivity in a double-blind, placebo-controlled trial of people with personality disorder taking lithium (Links, Steiner, Boiago and Irwin 1990), but lithium has considerable dangers when not taken as prescribed. Three randomized, double-blind placebo-controlled trials of fluoxetine (20–80 mg) are reported on in reviews by Solloff's (2000) and The American Psychiatric Association (2001) guidelines. The three trials show some support for efficacy on mood, anger and impulsivity but there are methodological limitations (Markowitz 1995; Salzman, Wolfson, Schatzberg et al. 1995; Coccaro and Kavoussi 1997). "Normal" volunteers taking paroxetine in a randomized double-blind placebo controlled study, had lower scores on hostility and negative affect compared with those on placebo (Knutson, Wolkowitz, Cole et al. 1998). Paroxetine, in a single, randomized, double-blind, placebo-controlled trial, resulted in a modest reduction of suicidal behavior in a group of patients with "repeated suicide attempts but not major depression" (Verkes, Van der Mast, Hengeveld et al. 1998). These results are consistent with the knowledge of people meeting diagnostic criteria for borderline personality disorder having diminished serotonergic function. These studies and early impressions from other SSRI trials are encouraging the consideration of SSRIs as a drug of first choice especially for impulsivity and affective dysregulation, if medication is being used. A medication response to SSRIs may occur as early as a few days but a trial should be at least 12 weeks (American Psychiatric Association 2001). Some clinicians hypothesie that SSRIs have an impact on inborn temperament, thereby assisting clients to use psychosocial treatments more effectively.

Neuroleptic agents

There have been double-blind placebo controlled trials of thiothixene, triflouperazine and haloperidol (Soloff 2000) and one double-blind trial of thiothixene and haloperidol (4–12 mg) (Serban and Siegel 1984) showing modest global improvement in symptoms. There has been one double-blind placebo controlled trial published to date using atypical antipsychotics. In this small study, olanzapine was associated with significantly greater changes compared to placebo on four of five subscales of the SCL-90 (Zanarini and Frankenberg 2001). In reviewing a number of studies using neuroleptic agents, Woo-Ming and Siever (1998) state, "... it may be reasonable to choose an antipsychotic medication for a borderline patient who has a predominance of psychoticlike features...". This is a position supported by The American Psychiatric Association (2001) guidelines. Because of their lower side effect profile, the newer antipsychotic agents (olanzapine, risperidone), are generally being used in clinical practice ahead of the older antipsychotics.

Anticonvulsants

Carbamazepine has been researched with mixed results with one study demonstrating improvement in impulsivity and dyscontrol (Gardner and Cowdrey 1986) but this was not replicated in a later study (Woo-Ming and Siever 1998). Sodium valproate has shown some early promise in open uncontrolled trials (Hollander 1999; Kavoussi and Coccaro 1998). In a randomized double-blind placebo control trial, clinicians rated clients diagnosed with borderline personality disorder treated with sodium valproate improving on measures of global symptoms and functioning compared with placebo (Hollander, Allen, Prieto-Lopez et al. 2001). However, the sample size was small, the drop out rate was high and there were no client administered ratings.

Older agents (tricyclic antidepressants, older MAOIs)

Some of the older noradrenergic agents can improve mood symptoms but sometimes worsen impulsivity, irritability and dyscontrol. This is in keeping with the theory that people meeting diagnostic criteria for borderline personality disorder have a dysregulated noradrenergic system. "Noradrenergic agents such as the tricyclic antidepressants or MAOIs are less desirable; although they may have an effect on depressive or atypical depressive features, results have been inconsistent in the trials so far. If they are used, patients should be carefully monitored for the appearance of increased impulsivity" (Woo-Ming and Siever 1998).

Other agents

Many other psychopharmacological agents have been reported to be successful in open uncontrolled trials or anecdotal case reports. Whilst the information from these sources may provide pointers for future research, they are short of the standard required to recommend treatment, especially in a client group whose symptoms naturally fluctuate. Of most interest are naltrexone (Bohus, Landwehrmeyer, Stiglmayr, Limberger et al. 1999; Links 1998; Roth, Ostroff and Hoffman 1996), clonidine, risperidone and clozapine (Benedetti, Sforzini, Colombo et al. 1998; Chengappa, Ebeling, Kang et al. 1999).

The prescribing clinician needs to resist the considerable pressure that often occurs for a quick cure. Prescribing needs to be done as one would for any other disorder with adequate doses taken consistently and for a satisfactory duration. Until this has taken place, the prescribing clinician needs to advise that the medication has not been adequately trialed and resist the pressure to change medication or add further medication. Prescribing clinicians need to integrate pharmacological and psychological effects such as the medication being experienced as a symbolic yet tangible currency of caring or authority. Also, clinicians need to prescribe in a manner which supports the notion that medication is an adjunct only to psychosocial treatment and affirms the client as the primary agent of change. Daily diarising of specific target behaviours of medication (e.g. psychotic-like features, depression, anxiety, irritability, sensitivity to feelings of rejection, self-harm, substance use, bingeing, quality of life, level of function) and medication side effects provides useful data in determining whether changes are related to medication or other variables.

In summary, if medication is to be used, fluoxetine or paroxetine will in general be a reasonable first choice especially for impulsivity and affective dysregulation. Dosages may need to be increased progressively to the higher range. In time, it is likely that other SSRIs will be shown to be effective. A neuroleptic agent could be a first choice if prescribing for someone with psychotic-like or psychotic symptoms or a history of psychotic symptoms. Mood stabilising medication such as sodium valproate is another possibility.

Prescribing in the acute situation

If a client can manage a crisis without external pharmacological assistance, this will greatly enhance their self-capacity and confidence for future crises. If this is not possible, the pragmatic use of minimal doses can de-escalate a crisis and stabilize the situation. The evidence base to recommend what medications to use is limited but sufficient for Soloff (2000) to state "The empiric literature supports the use of low-dose neuroleptics for the acute management of global symptom severity", a position supported by The American Psychiatric Association (2001) guidelines. Some people believe benzodiazepines to be contra-indicated in this client group because of their capacity to reinforce further crises, possible disinhibiting effect and potential for addiction. To use medication because of inadequate resources to provide psychosocial interventions is short of best practice.

In summary

- The term "borderline personality disorder" is unsatisfactory
- Point prevalence is about 1.8% of 19–55-year-olds
- People meeting criteria are well represented in mental health facilities, with estimates of 11% at community clinics and 20% in inpatient units
- High percentage of those attending drug and alcohol services meet criteria
- 75% are female

- 70% have a sexual abuse history
- 75% have a history of self-harm
- Borderline personality disorder might be best considered as severe personality difficulties rather than a discrete entity
- Diagnosis is multi-dimensional
- There is considerable overlap and comorbidity with other diagnoses
- Giving the client the "benefit of the doubt" and making a diagnosis of an Axis I disorder, till proven otherwise, may not always be in the interest of the client, as it might invite a client conceptualization that they are not responsible for their behaviour
- A positive diagnosis of borderline personality disorder ideally can be made without it being a diagnosis of exclusion or failure to respond to medications.
- Neurophysiology is characterized by reduced serotonergic activity
- A complex multifactorial aetiological model hypothesizes different individual pathways through the interaction of predisposing and resilience factors
- Long-term prognosis is reasonably good, provided people do not suicide
- Hospitalization has mostly ceased five years after first presentation
- Morbidity is high (self-harm, substance use, anxiety and depressive disorders, suicide)
- 46% have been victims of adult violence (rape – 31%, physically violent partner – 33%)
- Suicide rates range from 10–36%, depending on severity
- Health resource usage is high and drops considerably after effective treatment
- There is a paucity of treatment research to recommend evidence-based practice, so clinician focus has to be on best practice recommendations
- Commonalities between different models can guide best practice

- General mental health clinicians can provide effective treatment using general mental health skills. These skills include case management, crisis practice, skills training, rehabilitation and supportive psychotherapy
- The best researched psychosocial treatments for people with severe forms of the disorder are DBT, self psychology as carried out by Stevenson/Meares and psychoanalytic psychotherapy as reported on in a partial hospitalization program by Bateman and Fonagy
- Pharmacological treatment can have a limited role as an adjunct to psychosocial treatments

Part 2

Treatment issues and clinical pathways

Introduction

Effective treatment requires a skilled balance between encouraging client responsibility and autonomy, and offering clear supportive structures when needed. This section outlines how well-defined and well-supported roles for key clinicians and treatment teams can be developed in a system culture that minimizes burn-out and processes staff differences. Careful assessment, clinical plans and contracts encourage collaboration between clients and staff to improve client outcomes. Clinician empathy, validation and containment are imbedded in dealing with inevitable crises, which for the client, are an essential opportunity to practice dealing with distress. To enable hospitalizations to be brief requires clear understandings of issues around acute versus chronic suicidality and short versus long-term risks/gains. Skills development offers clients alternatives to self-harm and suicidality as ways of relieving internal distress and communicating to others. The principles of effective treatment outlined in this section can provide a foundation to firm up current skilful practice and address hurdles to effective treatments.

Assessment

The assessment provides the foundation for the clinical plan on which treatment will be based.

Assessment can be difficult given that interpersonal trust is damaged, but is crucial. An adequate assessment of a client's problems and needs is required for clinician and client to engage in a mutually

Treatment

Clinical Plan

Assessment

agreed upon plan of action. An unpleasant surprise awaits clinician and client when there is no initial assessment, and clinician and client proceed on a journey neither expect to be so eventful and traumatic. Having a thorough initial assessment assists all parties to engage and plan ahead realistically. The assessment will be modified according to the setting and context (whether in inpatient or outpatient settings, whether for crisis management or ongoing therapy and whether the client is well known to the clinician or not). Treatment issues exist right from the very beginning of an assessment. As such, gathering factual information needs to be balanced with other factors, such as the need to build a therapeutic alliance, motivation and commitment, to engage the client collaboratively, to instil realistic hope and to maximize client self-determination. This balance is seldom achieved in a first assessment. There is a danger, especially among inexperienced staff, of gathering information invasively which can complicate effective future treatment. This should not, however, be a reason to neglect doing a thorough risk assessment.

Assessment includes general information appropriate to any psychiatric assessment (i.e. demographic data, contact persons and social supports, presenting problem/s, stressors, risk assessment, level of function, past treatments, past psychiatric history, family psychiatric history, past medical history, current medications, drug and alcohol use, biographical history, temperament and personality style, mental status and diagnosis). This information should assist with confirming/disconfirming the diagnosis. Careful distinguishing of borderline personality disorder versus Axis I disorders is crucial to implementing effective treatment.

Further areas of assessment which may be needed include:

- Further risk assessment including determination of acute versus chronic suicidality (see rest of "Assessment" section and "The legal environment" section)
- Further mental status assessment including affect, presence of psychosis, and cognitive functioning
- Skills deficits and strengths, short and long-term levels of function, role function, role dysfunction and skills required

- Client goals and motivations for different types of treatment including effective and ineffective past treatments
- Family and/or current living environment (is this facilitating change and, if not, what else is required)
- Institutional/mental health system of care available to the client (is this facilitating change and, if not, what else is required)
- Personality style (including impulsivity, identity, anger, relationships, self-determination)
- How distress leads to current problem behaviours – behavioural chain analysis
- Formulation/Conceptualization: The brief synthesizing of pertinent information making linkages between present and past behaviours, feelings and events. This provides clarity and understanding as to how this person got to be who and where they are on the day of assessment. The conceptualization will underpin the clinical plan including targeting of skills acquisition and environmental change.
- Transition to treatment: This includes exploration of client, clinician and mutual goals; motivations of client and clinician and motivational interviewing. Out of this exploration a contract will generally evolve. Sometimes, however, there is not a matching of client and clinician goals or of how the goals will be achieved. In this case, the clinician does not give up on the client, but focuses on the advantages and disadvantages of contracting for treatment.

Motivation and commitment to change are areas of both assessment and treatment. Motivational interviewing was developed as an alternative in the substance use field to the "confrontation of denial" philosophy. Each client is recognized as possessing potential for change and it is the clinician's task to assist this manifesting. Clinicians take a warm interested "ally" stance raising questions and information. Motivational interviewing explores with the client their "stuckness" and the hurdles blocking them moving through the natural stages of change; precontemplation, contemplation, determination (commitment to action) and action (DiClemente 1991; Miller 1983; Miller and Rollnick 1991).

Commitment to change is dimensional, varying over time, depending on circumstances such as mental state and level of challenge. Early and ongoing attention to commitment may assist the client when circumstances get to feel "too hard". Commitment to treatment and change may be improved by increased awareness of the issues and the pros and cons of change, internal attribution of change, internal congruence as opposed to cognitive dissonance, client generated external rewards and an awareness of past gains made by commitment to change.

The table below provides a checklist for clinicians doing an assessment.

Assessment

Apart from the usual assessment, the following features need to be kept in mind:

Information gathering vs therapeutic alliance
(mindful of the balance)

Psychiatric history, including a thorough developmental history – as usually done

Skills
- Strengths/deficits – Skills required
- Levels of function – Consistency of levels of function (short and long-term)
- Role function/dysfunction (e.g. work, friend, family member)

Family/friends/social supports
- Currently helpful or not
- If not helpful – what needs to be considered?

Mental health care
- Currently helpful or not
- If not helpful – what needs to be considered?
  (past treatment history, especially patterns)

Relationship patterns (e.g. abusive partners; all-on-all-off; avoidant; based around substance use)

Personality style especially: Impulsivity, anger, identity, self-determination and relationships

Assessment (cont.)

Behavioural chain analysis – How distress or "triggers" leads to problem behaviours

Self-harm
- About suicide or not about suicide
- If not about suicide – does it decrease distress or is it "communication behaviour" (see "Self-harm" section)

Risk assessment (including acute vs chronic suicidality; short-term vs long-term risk)

Mental status especially:
- Affect
- Psychosis
- Cognitive functioning
- Therapeutic alliance (how are clinician and client getting on?)

Conceptualization/formulation
- Synthesis
- Linkages
- Patterns

Diagnosis
Comorbid diagnoses e.g.
- Major depression
- Substance use disorder

Goals
- Client
- Clinician
- Common Goals

Transition to treatment
- Treatment options
- Motivation for treatment – including different types and places of treatment
- Contracting
- Orientation to treatment

Risk assessment

Whilst statistical risk factors such as age, substance use and depression are useful, clinical decisions need to be very individualized. "Extreme caution is required when applying probabilities derived from actuarial methods to *individuals*" (Ministry of Health 1998).

Individualized risk assessment will be influenced by:

- Intensity of the emotional pain, especially feelings of hope, hopelessness and despair
- Whether the client can see alternatives
- Whether the client feels alienated (experiencing the availability of caring others, protective effects of connection)
- Client view of the "afterlife" (e.g. assumption that death will end the pain; reunited with a loved person)
- Degree of suicide planning
- Prior suicide attempts are correlated with later suicide (Tanney and Motto 1990)
- Aborted suicide attempts (where the person planned an attempt and at the last minute changed their mind) correlated with later suicide (Barber, Marzuk, Leon, Portera 1998)
- Distinguishing acute from chronic suicide patterns (see rest of "Assessment" section and "The legal environment" section)
- Short-term vs long-term risk/gain (see rest of "Assessment" section and "The legal environment" section)

Differentiating acute and chronic suicidal and self-harm patterns

A detailed history of past and current suicidality and self-harm will provide benchmark information required to develop a longitudinal treatment plan and to guide crisis treatments. One of the difficult aspects for clinicians is attempting to intervene appropriately when the client is suicidal or intends to self-harm. The question of the level of intervention that would be the most helpful is difficult. One method of managing this more predictably is for the assessment to include a very detailed history of the self-harm or suicidality, its antecedents and outcomes. If there is a long-standing pattern of behaviour and outcomes this could be labelled as a chronic pattern.

The treatment plan is then established, including the level of intervention considered to be most helpful both at times of non-crisis and at times of crisis. This treatment plan will be developed at non-crisis times allowing for time to debate areas of concern and the capacity to get wide support and cohesion amongst treating clinicians. The treatment plan will be reviewed by peers or supervisors to ensure it meets reasonable clinical standards. The treatment plan will have types and levels of intervention aimed at providing effective treatment and minimizing overall risk and will have taken into account short-term and long-term risk and gains of different interventions. This plan is negotiated with and made clear to the client. This method of using the chronic pattern as a benchmark for developing and carrying out longitudinal and crisis treatments needs to be widely supported at all levels and is discussed further in the next section on crisis assessment. The following is a guide for a longitudinal suicide and self-harm assessment. This should be done over several sessions as it is often very difficult for the client. The documentation should cover about 2–3 typed pages if it is thorough enough.

Longitudinal suicide and self-harm assessment

- History of suicide and self-harm behaviours, thoughts and feelings (incl. duration, long-term and current frequency, methods, intended and actual lethality [degree of injury, level of secrecy, OD doses])
- Known suicide and self-harm triggers
- Behaviour pattern leading to suicidality and self-harm
- Outcomes of suicidal and self-harm behaviours
- Behaviour pattern indicative of increased risk (need for risk assessment form)
- Past treatment strategies (include why some strategies have not been successful)
- Responses client reports as unhelpful
- Responses client reports as helpful
- Responses elicited from carers
- Function of self-harm
- Client skills/strengths

Crisis assessment

If a client has a well defined and documented chronic pattern of suicidality and self-harm and there is a proactively agreed plan around the level of support and intervention around crisis situations, then the type of intervention at a time of crisis could be determined by the presence or absence of a chronic pattern at the time of crisis. Each time the client presents, the appropriate assessment of behaviours, mental state and other risk factors is completed. If this fits the chronic pattern for the client and the interventions are documented in the treatment plan then the treatment plan stands. However, should the presentation be different to the usual presentation then the crisis worker should consider altering the interventions recommended in the treatment plan. Similarly if the mental state of the client is such that the client cannot be said to be responsible for their own behaviour then active intervention by the crisis worker should take place. Using the chronic pattern to guide crisis decision-making can be a robust method of providing effective treatment by managing the decision-making and appropriately tolerating at-risk behaviours and situations without resorting to interventions which could be harmful or unhelpful. Harmful interventions may include inappropriately restrictive, inconsistent or regression promoting interventions. This method needs to be supported by very good policies and procedures, peer and supervisory support, excellent team work, excellent system work, backing at the highest level and evidence at all levels of good clinical practice and documentation. In these circumstances often quite severe self-harm or suicidality can be treated successfully.

The format below is an example of how this assessment might be thought about and documented. The format is used with a close knowledge of the chronic pattern of this particular client.

Crisis risk assessment

Name_____   Date_____

Time_____

This risk assessment is to be completed by clinical staff at any time there is a noted change that indicates a possible change in the risk profile of the client

Context

Behaviour – Current
How is it different from chronic pattern?

Mood
How is it different from chronic pattern?

Affect (feeling state)
How is it different from chronic pattern?

Suicidal thinking (plans, context)
How is it different from chronic pattern?

Other thinking
How is it different from chronic pattern?

Engagability (eye contact, keeping promises, warmth, honesty)
How is it different from chronic pattern?

Perceptual changes
How is it different from chronic pattern?

Judgement
How is it different from chronic pattern?

Triggers/current stressors

Coping skills and ability to use them

Treatment plan review?   Yes   No

Next review (Date and Time)

Who will complete the next review

Signature of person completing this risk assessment

Date

Interventions

Client–clinician relationship

A desire for a solid, consistent, caring, enduring relationship is almost universal. People meeting diagnostic criteria for borderline personality disorder frequently have childhood and adult histories of relationships that have been notable for problems in attachment. Evidence-based treatments, and for that matter virtually all treatment schools, have a secure, firm, attached relationship with the therapist as central to the treatment.

This firm, attached relationship is not easy to establish and maintain for clinician and client alike. Fear of abandonment and difficulty being alone have been named as core client feelings (Gunderson 1996). It is common for clients to want more from their clinicians than clinicians can provide. This threatens the therapeutic relationship because of associated feelings of hurt, anger, disappointment, rejection and abandonment.

Without a sufficiently viable relationship, treatment will falter. Skills training and organizational structures, whilst important, will be insufficient if they are not integrated within a model which supports and values the centrality of the client–clinician relationship. This relationship, in turn, needs to be supported by the organization and includes supervision for the clinician.

Team/system culture

The culture ideally matters to the people who are part of it; people define themselves in terms of it, care about it, are willing to sacrifice to improve it and members seek to help weaker members. (Adapted and printed with permission from Gleisner S., personal communication 1997). The culture ideally is co-operative and mutually supportive; accommodates constructive conflict and is not divided by it; proactively addresses staff differences; validates the clients, the work and the clinicians doing the work (including the provision of adequate resourcing) and encourages and supports professionally indicated risk-taking (see "Professionally indicated risk-taking" section).

Clinical plan

> A significant turning point occurred when a group of mental health professionals began to meet and discuss how they could best deliver their services to develop my own coping skills whilst still leaving me feeling supported. At first I was sure these meetings were a conspiracy and when first presented with the notion of a clinical plan was dubious to say the least. Having a clinical plan completely changed the focus – no longer were others responsible for my life and safety. Instead I was responsible for my own feelings and subsequent actions. Prolonged admissions under the Mental Health Act were suddenly a part of my past and, while terrified, I quickly responded positively to the control I was now being handed.
>
> (Jackson 1999)

The importance of developing a clinical plan is highlighted by Kjelsberg, Eikeseth and Dahl's (1991) finding that the lack of a treatment contract was a significant predictive factor of suicide in people meeting diagnostic criteria for borderline personality disorder. Whilst the concept of developing, implementing and reviewing a clinical plan is obvious, processes and functional relationships required are challenging, sometimes to such a degree that an adequate plan does not exist. The importance of a clinical plan as the foundation of initial treatment, central to provision of ongoing effective treatment, cannot be overemphasized. Having a regularly reviewed clinical plan implies that individualized conceptualization/formulation of client issues take place, that relevant parties are participating in ongoing dialogue and are aware of and in reasonable agreement with the clinical plan. This will encourage integration of services and keep surprises to a minimum. Wherever possible, the plan is a mutual, collaborative endeavour between the client and the treating team, usually represented by the key clinician. The plan includes crisis guidelines, pathways to respite and hospitalization, and the client's individualized crisis strategies. The latter includes what has and has not worked in the past, including a list of safe people to contact, safe places to go to, activities which make the client feel safe, self-soothing skills, emotion acceptance skills and alternatives to self-harm. Possible templates of clinical plans are provided below.

CLINICAL PLAN
Administration

Clinical Plan updated on [   ]   Next update on (at least monthly) [   ]

Client contact details [   ]

This plan is known to [   ]

This plan is available to [   ]

Significant others contact details [   ]

Key Clinician [   ]

(outpatient clinician responsible for Clinical Plan development and integration of services)

Meetings scheduled [   ]

Backup for Key Clinician [   ]

Therapist (*if different from key clinician*) [   ]

Meetings scheduled [   ]

Prescribing clinician (*outpatient*) [   ]

Meetings scheduled [   ]

Other meetings scheduled (relatives/friends, GP, inpatient/crisis link person/s, child protection agency...)

[   ]

Inpatient Link Person
(*responsible for coordinating inpatient care and with key cllinician for inpatient entry and exit criteria and pathways*)

[   ]

Crisis Team Link Person
(*responsible for coordinating crisis care and with key cllinician for crisis care entry and exit criteria and pathways*)

[   ]

Link People for other services

[   ]

Clinical Overview

Summary of Psychatric History

Major Goal/s (*agreed upon by client and key clinician for next year - no more than 2*)

Lesser Goal/s

Stage of Treatment 1 Stabilization and safety   **Suicide Risk History**   1 Intermittentaly acute
                        2 Exploration/metabolism of trauma   2 Intermittentaly acute
                        3 Generalizing changes and finishing   superimposed on chronic
                                                                                       3 Chronic
                                                                                       4 Not current

Self-Harm   Method

                   Frequency

                   Purpose of self-harm (client and clinician views)

Summary of Current and Recent History (*stressors, issues, goals*)

Current Medication/s

Key Issues

Client attached to key clinician or therapist	yes/no	Relevent services in agreement with Clinical Plan	yes/no
Key Clinician empowered to determine treatment	yes/no	Supervision in place and meeting the need	yes/no
Relevent people aware of Clinical Plan	yes/no	Family/friends needs being met	yes/no

Crisis plan — clinician focused

(Clinician and client will have a copy of this and Crisis Plan — Client focused)

Pathway of agreed contact at time of crisis

9-5 Monday — Friday

Out of Hours

Key Clinician's Guidelines for crisis worker *(eg. strategies which help/don't help)*

Respite Plan *(incl.alternatives to hospitalization)*

Hospital Admission Plan

Crisis plan—client focused

(Client and clinician will have a copy of this and Crisis Plan — Clinician Focused)

People who stay alive generally do well!

The place of crisis in my healing

(e.g. a crisis can be helpful to me in the long term. How I can use a crisis to practise and consolidate new skills)

My Crisis Strategies:

Safety   Safe places

Safe people

Activities/Items which make me feel safe

Self Soothing Skills

Distress Reduction Skills

Emotion Acceptance Skills

Alternatives to Self-harm

Other Strategies

My pathway of agreed contact at time of crisis

9-5 Monday—Friday

Out of Hours

Inpatient plan

This inpatient plan is either:

A) **Client Controlled Admission**

B) **Limited transfer of treatment planning to the inpatient team (No changes made to medication, therapy etc. which remains responsibility of outpatient service.)**

C) **Larger transfer of treatment and treatment planning to the inpatient team**

Aftercare Plan (*incl. contract and pathway for future acute admission — to be worked on before admission*)

Key Clinician guidelines for inpatient plan (*strategies which help/don't help*)

Goal/s of Admission (*rarely more than 2, as contracted with client*)

Key Clinician/therapist can/can't see client during hospitalization

Meetings Scheduled

Inpatient Link Person

Prescribing Clinician

Key Clinician/therapist (*if in contract*)

Treatment monitoring and planning

Other

Length of Admission   Time and Date of return 'home'

Contracts (*incl. contigencies, if any, for self harm/suicide/homicide statements or behaviour*)

A fictitious example of a crisis plan

(including Hospitalization)
for A... and Goodenuf Mental Health Services

Introduction

A... meets diagnostic criteria for borderline personality disorder. She experiences frequent suicidality and has often self-harmed. The Crisis team provides a crisis response. I Listen provides therapy and IM Available is the key clinician. This plan is a unique individualized plan drawn up collaboratively by and for A... and Goodenuf Mental Health Services.

Note!

This plan assumes client is well known and issues of short-term vs long-term risk/gain have been explored. If client is not well known, err on the side of caution and get to know client exploring short-term vs long-term risk/gain. The plan also assumes a willingness to vigorously address acute suicidality if assessment of client indicates this.

Aims and duration of plan

To clarify Goodenuf Mental Health Services' roles in A...'s treatment.

The plan will be reviewed after one month or sooner if needed.

Consultation

The plan has been agreed to by Goodenuf's Community, Inpatient and Crisis Teams and been approved of by Dr. IM Important, Clinical Director, Goodenuf Mental Health Services.

The plan

1. I Listen (Therapist) will have weekly scheduled sessions with A

A fictitious example of a crisis plan *(cont.)*

2. IM Available (Key clinician) is available to meet with A... for support and crisis care during usual working hours.

3. Crisis and Emergency Services will be involved out of hours as follows:
   (a) Telephone and face to face supportive contact (see format over)
   (b) Assessments of Safety (see below)
   (c) Hospitalization when there is considered to be imminent risk of loss of life.
   (d) If A... has already self-harmed (not about suicide) – focus on immediate safety and appropriate medical care and keep contact brief whenever possible.
   (e) Staff will not act to prevent minor self-harm but will provide support to A... to help her deal with her feelings and the situation
   (f) Staff will not prescribe or dispense any medications. This task is organized by Dr. Clear (the designated prescribing clinician)

Please remember that an important part of this plan is consistency across services – deviations from the plan are deviations from a long-term treatment plan, which in turn, puts pressure on the service involved.

Note!

This plan assumes client is well known and issues of short-term vs long-term risk/gain have been explored. If client is not well known, err on the side of caution and get to know client exploring short-term vs long-term risk/gain. The plan also assumes a willingness to vigorously address acute suicidality if assessment of client indicates this.

Adapted and reprinted with the permission of Balance, Auckland Healthcare

A fictitious example of a crisis plan *(cont.)*

Supportive contact

The premise of phone support is that self-harm/suicidality is a solution to the problem of how A...feels. The goal is to find other solutions to cope with the feelings

1. Scheduled phone calls by crisis worker every...day/s – 15 minutes (if possible). You may need to negotiate when you could call back
2. Listen supportively – A's distress is real
3. Try wherever possible to focus on solutions to problem other than suicide/suicide thinking
4. Discuss feelings in context of chain of precipitating events – Summarize
5. Review how she has already tried to cope. Helpful activities are: *(e.g. talking to a friend, taking a shower, gardening.)*
6. In the last five minutes of the call ask her for advice about what she could do to cope with how she is feeling. Be cautious about giving advice!
7. A focus for A... will be how she will get through to the next scheduled appointment
8. Further phone calls should be by A... calling us prn – not scheduled calls from us

Safety assessment

A... chronically experiences a level of suicidality. Normal principles of risk assessment apply but note:

1. Hospitalization is only to prevent suicide or life-threatening self-harm or to provide brief predetermined time out.
2. Don't ask A... to guarantee her safety – This is not a sensible proposition for her.
3. Remember that living with some risk is a difficult and everyday part of A...'s life – and will also be a part of ours.

Adapted and reprinted with the permission of Balance, Auckland Healthcare

A fictitious example of a crisis plan (cont.)

Hospitalization

(a) Hospitalization is only to prevent suicide or life-threatening self-harm or to provide brief predetermined time out

(b) If no inpatient beds are available, arrange alternative only if the safety focus can be maintained

(c) Hospitalizations are short (12–72 hours)

(d) The focus of care is to ensure safety or in the case of time out, a friendly, courteous but relatively neutral relationship

(e) Discussions with A... can be about the feelings and events leading up to the lack of safety and things the client can do to decrease distressing feelings. Don't get drawn into providing therapy or treatment issues beyond the immediate limited focus of the hospitalization

(f) Review and adjustment of the community generated clinical plan is the task of the community team. This includes medication, involvement of significant others and other treatment issues

(g) It is likely that A... will still be experiencing a level of risk to safety upon discharge

Signed A...
Key Clinician ....
Community Mental Health Manager...
Dr. IM Important, Clinical Director...
Plan ratified by the complex borderline syndrome review forum
(or other peer review meeting) on ....

Feedback

Is this working? Feedback to IM Available (Key Clinician) or Dr IM Important

Adapted and reprinted with the permission of Balance, Auckland Healthcare

Duration of treatment

The best studies of outpatient treatment with people meeting diagnostic criteria for severe forms of borderline personality disorder had people in treatment for one year (Linehan *et al.* 1991; Stevenson and Meares 1992). Whilst positive results were obtained during this duration, both groups see best practice treatment lasting longer than this, perhaps on average 2–4 years. Some clients, like the "butterfly" clients described by Linehan (1993a), flit in and out of treatment and cannot initially be engaged successfully in consistent regular long-term treatment, but can be engaged in "long-term intermittent treatment". Here, an individual clinician or system will be available to the client if/when they seek crisis or short-term treatment. The principle is to maintain what advantages of continuity are possible and for the client to feel connected and not abandoned. It is easier to maintain an optimistic position that is so necessary for positive outcome, if a long-term perspective (years) is held.

Prioritizing interventions

People meeting diagnostic criteria for borderline personality disorder frequently present unremittingly with a wide range of important pressing problems, which are potentially overwhelming for client and clinician. This presents the clinician with a dilemma of what to focus on. Many authors have broken down therapy into different stages (Briere 1992; Herman 1992; Linehan 1993a). Herman (1992) describes a three-stage model with the first stage being about stabilization, safety and trust, the second stage about emotionally expressive work (including direct exploration of trauma material) and the third stage about generalization of changes into the wider community of the client. Whilst presented in a linear fashion, this three stage model, involves considerable movement between stages as the person's life circumstances and internal well-being fluctuate. Most of the difficulties experienced in this work are in the first stage, which needs to be accordingly given high value and status. Treatment priorities in Stage 1 will be guided by the principle of doing what is going to best achieve stabilization and safety. Clearly acute suicide interventions take priority, as would, for example, life-threatening weight loss in someone with anorexia nervosa. A client who is using heroin daily, and committing crimes to sustain the drug habit, is likely to be assisted towards stabilization by getting onto a regular consistent dose of methadone. Other examples of activities which might best assist stabilization include developing a clear, coherent clinical plan or tending to the client's accommodation needs. The prioritizing needs to be individualized to the particular situation each client is in.

DBT (Linehan 1993a) uses a similar prioritizing process as follows:

Pre-treatment Stage
– Assessment, commitment to and orientation to therapy
Stage 1
– Suicide and self-harm behaviours
– Therapy interfering behaviours (of client or clinician. e.g. client not coming to sessions, clinician resentment towards the client)
– Quality of life issues (e.g. disabling anxiety, limited relationship skills)
Stage 2 – Posttraumatic stress therapy

Sexual abuse needs to be recognized and its importance acknowledged. There is expert consensus that specific psychological exploration of abuse material should only be done when there is sufficient stabilization. Briere (1992) writes of the need to balance consolidation vs exploration. Understandably, inexperienced therapists, recognising the aetiological importance of the abuse, may enter into psychological exploration too early, causing destabilization.

Staging treatment

Stage One	Stage Two	Stage Three
Stabilization, Consolidation, Safety	Emotional exploration	Generalization

Empathy and validation

Clients generally have had lifetime histories where their emotional experience of the world has not been understood. At times, they have had their personal experiences minimized, criticized or disbelieved. The impact of living with such devaluation and invalidation, during the formative years of childhood, leads to major problems in all areas of life. Clinicians need to find ways to be as empathic as possible with clients' experience, which is not always easy to achieve.

Empathy requires the clinician to attempt to get close to knowing the experience of the client. This requires listening to the client as free from preconceptions as possible and to "suspend judgement about the contents of the mind" in the "service of discovery" (Marguiles 1984). Effective treatment, of course, requires clinicians to "strive for a position of tension between knowing and not-knowing" (Marguiles 1984).

Care of nurses on acute inpatient units has been categorized according to different levels of care from the least helpful to the most helpful: belittlement; contradicting the client; offering platitudes; providing solutions without options; solutions with options; affective involvement which expresses concern and addresses client's feelings; affective involvement with options given to the client (Gallop, Lancee and Garfinkel 1989; Lancee, Gallop, McCay and Toner 1995). Lancee *et al.* (1995) found that "For impulsive patients, only one limit-setting style – affective involvement plus offering options – kept anger at a low level". In other words, empathy, validation and a solution focus.

Validation as described by Linehan (1993a) has similarities to empathy and invites a more active clinician component, as well. The clinician will look for that part of the client's experience that is valid and share this with the client. The stance is that current client experiences and behaviours are perfectably understandable considering biology, past experiences and current circumstances. The client is assumed to be doing the best they know how. Validation is balanced with challenge to change. The clinician is also invited to encourage or "cheerlead" the client. This aspect of validation, which is future focused, is about the clinician's belief in the client's capacity to achieve goals and change.

Both empathy and validation aim to accept the client as they are and encourage the client to empathize with and validate themselves, so that they can internalize the process.

Containment/holding

The concepts of "holding" and "containment" are important in determining priorities. Containment is a metaphor used to describe activity that assists feelings to be experienced in a manner that is constructive. That is, feelings are "held" within the "container". Both psychodynamic ("working through") and cognitive-behavioural ("exposure") treatments place emphasis on the therapeutic importance of experiencing affect. However, both schools of treatment recognize that the experiencing of affect has the potential to be overwhelming, leading to a deterioration and hence the importance of "containment" and "holding".

Containment/holding

Containment

The capacity to hold feelings without engaging in behaviours we are likely to regret

We know

People learn best when affect is present provided this affect is not overwhelming

The problem

To deal with overwhelming affect, we engage in survival behaviours, which we might later regret

The behaviours meet a short-term need at the expense of long-term function

The tasks

The task is to experience as much affect as possible provided this is not overwhelming

Containment/holding *(cont.)*

The client, clinician, treatment team, supervisor and the organization all have important roles in maximizing holding/containing

When affect is potentially overwhelming, the task is to find and engage in constructive behaviours that will enable the affect to not be overwhelming, that is, to be contained

Such behaviours are holding or containing behaviours

Containing behaviours

Containment includes people feeling safe, supported and valued

Containment includes clarity of boundaries and expectations

Containment includes having a treatment plan and a structured philosophy of treatment

Containment may include structured activity such as a scheduled telephone call or it might be a process of being calm, fully present and attentive

"Holding in supportive psychotherapy involves the capacity to 'do nothing', simply to be with the patient within the confines of the therapeutic frame, providing a still point in a chaotic world of illness and struggle" (Holmes 1995).

Transitional people and items

As described in the section "Client–clinician relationship", effective treatments are based on a secure attached client–clinician relationship. This necessary attachment, however, has its own inevitable problems when the clinician is not available in the way that the client would like.

In exploring and balancing client needs with therapist availability, Gunderson (1996; 2001) lists a "hierarchy of transitional options for use during therapist absences" from most soothing to least soothing. These are:

- ◆ Therapist accessible by phone (as needed, scheduled)
- ◆ Colleague cover (as needed, scheduled)
- ◆ Therapist associated transitional objects (tape, note, item)
- ◆ Non-therapist transitional items (friends, events).

The choice of transitional options will be determined by the often-competing principles of maximum self-sufficiency and holding/containment. In general, the therapist's task is to maximize self-sufficiency by using the least containing option possible to sustain a viable therapeutic relationship, and to then move to less containing, more self-sufficient options as the client progresses.

Self-harm

It's all my fault ... I always end up destroying people because I need more than they can give ... I am just warped forever ... The damn world doesn't want me. I just don't fit with the rest of the world ... Maybe if I hurt myself it will lessen the pain. A minute later I walked into the women's bathroom and slit my side with a razor blade, making a very superficial cut at first, then cutting deeper and deeper. As I started to cut, the physical pain and blood became a welcome distraction. As I cut deeper ... my mind began to feel relieved of the torment. My body eased of the tension and I began to feel comforted.

(Leibenluft, Gardner and Cowdry 1987;
Reprinted with the permission of Guilford Press)

I took the hammer and hit my arms over and over again, but couldn't seem to break them. The numbness was in my head, ears roaring. I felt no pain. I got angry at myself for not being able to break my arm. Then I grabbed the hammer and started on my legs from knee to hip, hitting myself over and over, first on the one leg, and then the other .... The numbness was taking over.

(Leibenluft, Gardner and Cowdry 1987;
Reprinted with the permission of Guilford Press)

I quickly discovered my incredible need, or perceived need, to be cared for and helped would be met by professionals if I self-harmed, or threatened to self-harm. This was in no way an attempt to manipulate or dramatize. My coping skills were severely lacking, if they had ever existed, and I was genuinely unable to tolerate the incredible pain I felt

(Jackson 1999)

Persistent self-harm is frequently associated with the diagnos borderline personality disorder and includes cutting, burning, bruising and overdosing. It is critical to be clear, cross-sectionally and longitudinally, whether actions of harming the body were intended to suicide or for other reasons. Self-harm most commonly is used to alleviate emotional distress especially related to anxiety and anger. In these situations self-harm is a private act. A biological theory, which has some research support (Links 1998) hypothesizes self-harm releasing endogenous opiates, which makes the person feel better, like injecting heroin. Psychological processes are listed below in the table "Reasons for self-harm".

Reasons for self-harm

Internal process

Distress reduction (especially anger and anxiety)
To gain control over own inner experiences
Distraction
To replace an emotional pain with a physical pain
To make the emotional pain tangible and concrete
To maintain sense of integration (Feel alive, centred and grounded. Not disintegrated or "falling to pieces")
To express anger towards emotional self (punish self)
To express hate towards body (punish self)
To prevent dissociation
To cause dissociation

Communication behaviour

To feel heard
To communicate the intensity of subjective distress
To elicit behaviours from others which will decrease the pain/distress (attempt to get needs met. e.g. partner comes back, admission to hospital)
To express anger to others

In most of these instances a mind-body split or negative body image enables the body to be sacrificed to meet emotional goals.

Suicide

Successful treatment will lead to more adaptive alternatives of dealing with emotional distress. Treatment may involve a behavioural chain analysis of the sequence of events leading to self-harm, with the intention of the client becoming more aware of possible points to intervene differently in the future. (see section "Behaviour chain and solution analysis – fictitious clinical vignette 1 and 2"). This is a core feature of cognitive behavioural treatment approaches including DBT. The earlier in the pathway the intervention, the better. Frequently however, especially with clients new to treatment, interventions may only be able to be carried out immediately before self-harm or not at all.

Immediate alternatives to self-harm include activities that are somewhat less harmful, distracting activities and self-soothing activities. Determining the precise reason for self-harm with each individual on each occasion is essential in guiding treatment strategies. Usually clients can at least identify that they self-harmed to deal with unwanted distress, which provides a starting point to determining and naming what this distress was.

Self-harm actions which are covert communications are generally of more emotional difficulty for clinicians. Whilst self-harm as communication behaviour comprises a minority of self-harm, it represents much of what clinicians see, because obviously the intention is that the self-harm is visible. Here, the clinician will attempt to encourage overt communication alternatives and not reinforce the communication behaviour.

Where self-harm is about relief of internal distress, many clinicians ascribe to a harm-reduction model. This model sees self-harm as a means the client has developed, although far less than ideal, to deal with distress.

> Self-injury is a fundamentally adaptive life preserving coping mechanism. It enables people with overwhelming and often undifferentiated affect, intense psychological arousal, intrusive memories, and dissociative states to regulate their experiences and stay alive.
>
> (Connors 1996)

The task is to develop alternative ways of dealing with the distress. Whilst these skills are developing, a harm-reduction model encourages the person, if they are going to self-harm, to do so in a manner less likely to be life-threatening, disfiguring, or causing permanent damage. Some examples include using ice to distract or cause pain instead of cutting, cutting the body in safe places which will not easily be visible in the future; avoiding tendons, arteries and nerves; cutting as superficially as possible; using clean razor blades; not sharing razor blades and cutting in a manner which will result in less scarring. Other examples include avoiding self-harm which requires a person arriving at a certain time in order to not die and being knowledgable about the pharmacology of medications used in overdosing, where the purpose of the overdose is to temporarily blot out emotional pain.

It is preferable to intervene as early as possible in the chain of events leading to self-harm. This may be beyond the skills of the client especially initially in treatment. The table below lists some activities which might prevent self-harm just prior to the self-harm occurring.

Interrupting self-harm pathway just prior to self-harm

Physical activity (these activities may also be grounding, pleasurable, symbolic or distracting)

Going for a walk/run, digging in the garden, housework, martial arts, punching pillow

Distraction (may also be grounding or pleasurable)

Reading a book, cooking, working, going to a movie, snapping an elastic band on skin, holding ice cubes

Grounding

Going for a walk/run, digging in the garden, touching the soil, smelling flowers and plants

Pleasurable activities (may also be distracting or grounding)

Interrupting self-harm pathway just prior to self-harm (cont.)

Going for a walk/run, digging in the garden, reading a book, cooking, going to a movie, having a bath

Symbolic or simulation

Cutting meat specially kept in the fridge/freezer, drawing red marks on skin, drawing on paper, poetry, journal, punching pillow, tearing up paper, breaking own cheap crockery without scaring anyone

The exercise in the table below on "Self-exploration of reasons for self-harm" is intended to assist readers to understand why people self-harm and to decrease the distance between clients and clinicians. It is included in its current format in response to workshop participants to have a copy of the exercise as they experienced it.

Self-exploration of reasons for self-harm

The exercise has been adapted and printed with permission from Williams O., Workshop – 1997, One Body at Risk – Keeping the Client Safe

Introduction

We encourage the exercise to be used in a manner which is safe for participants; inviting their consideration and capacity to choose to not engage in the activity, especially if they are not feeling centred and in a place of well-being. The activity for obvious reasons can trigger considerable feelings which participants need to be reminded about. We also suggest that participants pick an activity that is as minor as possible. In this context, the exercise is intended to be an educational one, not a therapeutic one. We let participants know that they will not be sharing their experience with anyone and the experience will be entirely internal. It is intended that in an educational workshop context this creates some safety.

Self-exploration of reasons for self-harm (cont.)

Purpose

The purpose of the activity is to explore reasons why people self-harm and to decrease the distance between our clients and ourselves.

Guided visualization exercise

Think of an activity where you self-harm – That is, an activity you engage in, which meets a short-term need but is something you regret doing in the long run. Examples might be cigarettes, alcohol, chocolate bars, not exercising, too much exercising, staying up late at night. Pick an activity which is more down the minor end ...

- What do I gain from this activity?
- The instant before I carry out the activity – What do I feel?
- The instant I have done the activity – What do I feel?
- How did I learn to do this?
- Where did I learn to do this?
- If I told the average person about this – What reaction could I expect?
- Do I feel I could live without doing this?
- What would I lose if I stopped doing it?
- What would I gain if I stopped doing it?
- Do I want to stop doing it?
- What do I need to do to stop doing it?

The first three questions focus on self-reflection or behavioural analysis and the last five questions on motivational issues, finishing with a question focused on solutions.

For the treating team there needs to be a very detailed analysis of the timing, antecedents, and situations in which self-harm takes place. As ambivalence is one of the core features of the presentation to clinical staff, the level of knowledge that the clinician has will be crucial to the appropriate intervention. This will mean that the issue can be explored in more depth, and that the client can be supported to become more aware of the precise nuances of their feeling states and therefore move towards intervening themselves. The treating team can also be actively looking at the contingencies operating that keep the self-harm alive inadvertently. Examples of this operating are that the client cannot get access to treatment or even a sympathetic ear unless self-harm has taken place. A phone call by the clinician in the later afternoon to the client may prevent the client accessing after-hours staff in a less healthy way.

Contracts

Contracts are frequently used and have an important role to play. Advantages of contracts are that:

- The parties have been talking to one another
- Mutual collaboration and power-sharing are implied with inappropriate power differences decreased
- Clients may feel empowered and therefore more in control
- Expectations and responsibilities are clarified (decreases idealization/devaluation and likelihood of complaints)
- Structure, predictability and a reality base are provided
- Self-control is increased because of clarity and structure
- A place of agreement is established that can be returned to when conflict arises

Some dangers of contracts are that they can be:

- One-sided
- Used as punishment
- Seen as a substitute for treatment (Miller, Eisner and Allport 1990).

As with joint ventures in any context, outcome is significantly determined by the degree of respect each party has for the other, the balance of power and the participation, investment and "buy in" of all parties.

> Creating a contract with a client is a reflection of the therapeutic relationship and is therefore only as good as the alliance on which it is founded. Whether a contract serves as a helpful adjunct to treatment

or as a counter therapeutic distancing device, depends on how it is conceptualized, designed and negotiated

(McMahon and Milton 1999)

The basis of a contract needs to be one of warmth, and goodwill towards the client with therapeutic gain in mind. The client must view it positively. Implied in the contract is a two sided negotiation about what the client can expect from the treating team and individuals within it as well as what the client agrees to. Any contract which just sets out a set of expectations around the behaviour expected of the client, is likely to be unhelpful and may be punitive. Should there be a temptation to produce such a document, a careful examination of the dynamic in the group should be undertaken to ensure the clinicians feelings are not getting in the way of good treatment.

There may be other types of contracts, which are between staff from a number of agencies which would be more like a memorandum of understanding which would delineate the roles and responsibilities of each of the agencies of staff. This is helpful in creating a shared and clear understanding of the roles of various parties.

Crisis work

Why crisis work as a core focus?

- ◆ Crises are central to the disorder and central to treatment
- ◆ The major difficulties in treatment are inevitably around crises
- ◆ Once crises are not occurring the client is over the most difficult period
- ◆ Crises are inevitable and necessary (This view decreases disappointment, frustration and clinician burn-out)
- ◆ Crises are essential to practise dealing with distress, a core feature of treatment
- ◆ Crisis work has not been linked with high status and value. This devalues this most important and difficult area of work

Crisis work is an important adjunct to core community treatment and will be guided by the clinical plan set out by the key clinician and client in consultation with the crisis team (see section "Clinical plan"). This written plan will be available to crisis workers, who will be especially interested in the client's prioritized crisis intervention options and how to best support these. Crisis workers will contribute to improving and modifying the evolving clinical plan. Crisis work will be problem and solution-focussed with clients encouraged to use skills they have been learning, especially those listed in their crisis plan. This will be balanced with empathic listening. Crisis work may include tending to the anxiety of significant people and organizations.

Frequently, crisis (and inpatient) services are treating people due to the absence of a comprehensive outpatient service, which is short of best practice.

> The failure to develop appropriate comprehensive programs within public mental health services for patients with BPD means that, despite considerable evidence that inpatient care is neither economically nor clinically effective, patients are treated in this sub-optimal alternative.
> (O'Brien and Flote 1997)

Crisis work with people meeting diagnostic criteria for borderline personality disorder is very different from the long-term engagement of the key clinician and therapist. The goal is to assist the person to get back to their pre-crisis level of function and to "live to fight another day". Crises are inevitable and an essential learning opportunity for the client to develop a more adaptive repertoire of responses. The crisis session needs to be structured, with goals of the session collaboratively defined, directing/redirecting discussion to the original problem and defined goals of the session and with clear roles and responsibilities. If an impasse is reached, the clinician can point out the impasse and consequences of certain behaviours, take time out and get a second opinion.

For many clients the crisis time is after-hours, when the usual services that support them are not available. Clients are tired and often more vulnerable at this time. It is essential that after-hours staff are well integrated into the treatment planning. They can offer a strong ally to the client when used well. For crisis workers not to feel overburdened with extra work or to feel they will be left to manage alone, they need to have clear up to date individualized clinical guidelines to work within.

Wherever possible, the clinician will avoid taking responsibility for the client, and involve the client in determining options. Crisis workers need to be supported and encouraged to take professionally indicated risks (see section "Professionally indicated risk-taking"), to tolerate high levels of anxiety associated with at-risk behaviours and to be aware of any client-controlled admission policy the system has (see section "Client-controlled brief acute admissions"). Clinicians need to be trained in and aware of the clinical and medicolegal issues around acute vs chronic suicidality and balancing short-term vs long-term risk/gain (see sections "Assessment", "Pragmatic conceptual frameworks guiding treatment" and "The legal environment"). Additional information which can be helpful in crisis work are available in sections under the following titles: risk assessment, crisis assessment, clinical plan, contracts, medicolegal risk, pharmacological treatment, duration of treatment, prioritising interventions, some anti-suicide interventions, crisis hierarchy, self-harm, limit-setting, acute inpatient services and client controlled brief acute admission.

Regression at times of crisis

Regression at times other than crises may be a carefully, collaboratively planned and appropriate therapeutic endeavour. At times of crisis, however, the regressed part of the person needs to be validated but, in general, not encouraged. The goal in the crisis situation is not primarily to grow through the process of regression, but to "live to fight another day" without further deterioration.

Some clients warm to the concept of "The Child Within" which clinicians need to respect and, if appropriate, acknowledge. Hearing and relating respectfully to the child dimension may enable that part of the person to feel heard. Having been heard, the child dimension might feel OK about valuing and encouraging their adult dimension. In a crisis situation this may enable the client to return to adult levels of functioning. Timing of the intervention is critical. Moving too fast, before the person feels sufficiently heard and responded to, could encourage further regression. On the other hand, moving too slowly may exhaust the resources available (associated with negative consequences for the client) or reinforce regression.

Which level of functioning to address and for how long is a professional judgement, guided by knowledge of the client. The clinician might consider movement in the following direction indicative of a shifting of relating from the child to the adult dimension in an evolving fashion:

1. "I can see you are in lots of pain. How can I help?" (this might speak to and imply some capacity to help the child dimension of the person)
2. "What can we do?" (begin attempt to speak to adult dimension of the person implying that both clinician and client have capacity to help)
3. "What are your options?" (attempt to speak to the adult dimension, which is the part that has the capacity to help)
4. "What can you do?"
5. "What are you going to do?"

Fictitious clinical vignette

You work in a community mental health clinic and most of the time have clients booked back to back. At the end of a routine session with you, despite your best efforts, your client remains in a very regressed state. It is 2 pm. She goes to the waiting room intending to get a cup of tea. At 4.30 pm. she is curled up in the corner unable to speak much. You are able to ascertain that she is not acutely suicidal. The clinic is due to close at 5pm, you are aware that her clinical plan involves avoidance of admission except for severe, acute suicide risk. You can't have enough of a conversation with her to get informed consent for anything.

Some anti-suicide interventions

The risk assessment will guide anti-suicide interventions, which may include:

◆ Instillation of realistic hope
◆ Looking for alternatives (problem definition and then a solution focus)
◆ Making connection and tending to client's feelings of alienation

- Looking for internal contradictions and ambivalence regarding desire to die. (Is there even a tiny part that doubts, that is fearful of dying, that objects to dying?) Heightening ambivalence. Getting client's internal commitment to engage in internal and external dialogue over this ambivalence
- Decreasing impulsivity by internal agreement to wait till next appointment to discuss ambivalence
- Create distance, if possible, from client's access to lethal weapons and drugs

Instillation of hope has similarities to Linehan's (1993a) concept of "cheerleading".

> Imagine that you have just been in a terrible earthquake. Huge buildings have crashed down. Fires are all around. Police, firefighters and construction workers are overtaxed, and no one is available to help you. The child you love most in the world is still alive, but trapped in a small space under a building. There is a tiny opening she could crawl through to escape if she could get to it, or, if she could move just 2 feet closer to the opening, you could grab her and pull her out. The opening is too small for you to crawl in and get her. Time is of the essence because a loudspeaker truck just went by telling everyone to clear the area; when the next aftershock comes, more of the building will fall down. You search for a stick or something to throw to her to grab hold of, with no success. The child is crying for help. She can't move because every one of her bones are broken! You can't reach her if she doesn't move. Would you decide that she is manipulating you or just being obstinate? Would you sit back and wait for her to move, reasoning that when she wants to get out she will? Probably not. What would you do? Cheerlead. Cry out, command, yell, cajole, sweet-talk, insist, plead, suggest, threaten, direct, distract – all of these, in proper context and with proper modulation of tone, are methods of cheerleading.
>
> (Reprinted with the permission of Guilford Press)

Acute inpatient services

> I had over 50 admissions to various psychiatric units over a 10 year period, some of which were brief but the majority lasting weeks to several months. I can now see that this was a destructive path, only serving to prove to me that I really was helpless and hopeless. I read

recently someone saying "If you live with the lame you learn to limp". I certainly believe that was true for me.

Hospital became a place which was too safe, where I took no responsibility for my self and had no need to take control of my life. This fed my belief that I was inadequate and unable to cope with life. The more my needs were met in hospital, the less I believed I could manage my own life. This led to an increased frequency and duration of admissions, leading me to believe I was getting 'sicker', thereby needing more help etc. etc – a never ending cycle of helplessness and hopelessness.

(Jackson 1999)

Acute inpatient services are an important part of coherent, coordinated clinical plans of service delivery but are an adjunct only to the comprehensive outpatient service provided. Acute inpatient services are not designed to provide ongoing treatment for people meeting diagnostic criteria for borderline personality disorder, yet frequently end up doing so by default, due to the absence of comprehensive outpatient services. There is consensus expert professional opinion that acute inpatient units can cause iatrogenic deterioration due to a culture and inherent structures that do not always encourage clients to maximize their self-sufficiency. Clients are sending out the same message,

The most important thing is, do not hospitalize a person with borderline personality disorder for any more than 48 hours. My self-destructive episodes – one leading right into another – came only after my first and subsequent hospital admissions, after I learned the system was usually obligated to respond. The least amount of ill-placed reinforcement kept me going. It prevented me from having to make a choice to get well or even finding out that I wasn't as helpless as I believed myself to be. ... I would never have the life I have today if I had continued to get the intermittent reinforcement of hospitalization.

(Williams 1998)

Alternatively, the client may demand discharge, whilst behaving in a manner which makes discharge a clinical dilemma (O'Brien 1998).

Common reasons for acute inpatient admissions are treatment of comorbid diagnoses, acute suicidality and respite to achieve stabilization. If admission is being considered for respite, it is best to aim towards creative alternatives, which maximize client self-determination, autonomy and responsibility. These include intensive outpatient support, domestic help, day stays, motels and supported accommodation. When they do occur, admissions need to be, wherever possible, brief (up to 72 hours) and focused on reducing symptoms related to the current crisis. The inpatient service needs to have clear structures with clinicians having clearly defined roles. A goal-focused contract needs to exist with, wherever possible, a clear discharge date and outpatient contract. Outpatient planning, which is at least as important as the inpatient "work", needs to be coordinated with and influenced by the key outpatient clinician and needs to have begun prior to admission. A contract with clearly defined readmission criteria and pathways to be readmitted needs to be in place preferably before admission or as soon as possible after admission. These robust structures provide the client and staff with a "greater sense of control and empowerment" (Milton and McMahon 1999).

Cognitive-behavioural programs using and modifying DBT methods have been developed for use on acute inpatient units (Miller *et al.* 1994; Milton and McMahon 1999) providing a clear structure for client and staff alike. Chain analysis of current behaviour and discussion of skills used can be part of the inpatient culture and implemented at times of distress and crisis.

Keeping acute admissions brief requires clear understandings of the issues of acute versus chronic suicidality, short vs long-term risk/gain (see section on "Assessment" and the section on "The legal environment"), and organizational support for professionally indicated risk-taking (see "Professionally indicated risk-taking" section). Involuntary admissions need to be avoided, wherever possible, (see "Clinical appropriateness of the use of mental health legislation" section) and lengthy admissions in an acute psychiatric unit subject to routine local peer review. Pre-discharge deterioration is a likely possibility. Discharging a client from hospital frequently involves some continuing risk. A professional risk–benefit analysis will determine whether staying in hospital is a greater or lesser risk. Brief acute admissions also require comprehensive community treatment programs that are seen by clients as desirable.

Many of the principles used with client-controlled admissions can be used in clinician-controlled admissions, if it is decided that the acute unit is a place of respite and not "treatment" (see section "Client-controlled brief acute admissions"). In units where brief admissions are proactively contracted for and able to be sustained, staff morale is higher with more positive attitudes to the clients involved.

Advantages and disadvantages of brief hospitalization

Potential advantages of brief hospitalization

Prevent suicide/homicide
Provide stability to enable aftercare plan to be set up
Respite to prevent deterioration
Treat comorbid diagnoses; psychosis/depression/
anorexia nervosa

Potential disadvantages of brief hospitalization

Increased regression
Decreased autonomy
Increased passivity
Hospital as rescuer
Institutional rules often increase power struggle
Contagion effect
- If identity is "self-harmer" – being the best "self-harmer"
- More extreme behaviours to compete for staff time
- Learned behaviour (Ex-consumers have described the profound impact that saying you are going to kill yourself has on the environment)
- Behaviours learned from other clients – e.g. that self-harm is effective in dealing with internal distress or influencing the external environment

General principles of brief hospitalization

Place of respite or treatment change?

- Decide whether the admission is for respite or treatment change

Short admission (6–72 hours)

Goals (clearly defined and regularly reviewed)

- Indicative of collaborative engagement with client (wherever possible)
- Helps set limits
- Helps decrease expectations, transference, regression, staff anger and frustration

Staff

- Staff (inpatient and community) have realistic expectations of inpatient staff
- Clearly defined roles and clearly defined lines of responsibility

Communication channels

- Communication system generally in place
- Establish/maintain information flow between all staff about this client

Ward culture

- Consider the philosophy that therapy happens in the community – staff are warm and helpful but do not attempt to treat underlying issues
- Least restrictive possible
- Positive reinforcement
- Encouragement of staff expressing different views (cohesion)
- Maximizing matching of staff and clients
- Managing rather than encouraging regression
- In some circumstances, a high amount of structure initially lessening towards discharge
- Maximize client responsibility

General principles of brief hospitalization *(cont.)*

Aftercare plans

- From beginning of admission, plan for return home (discharge)
- An adequate aftercare plan is as important as settling the crisis
- Aftercare plans include stability of client, client's support system and client's key clinicians
- Relapse planning (prevention)
- Readmission criteria and procedures to be followed, known to relevant people

Contingencies

- Proactive with contingencies if/when plan comes unstuck

Frequent review

- Repeated review of the clinical plan
- Amounts of dependency, structure and responsibility
- Behaviours to positively reinforce

Stabilize client's community network

- Encourage client to maintain connections with their significant people
- Stabilize client's community treatment network if community team have been unable to achieve this
- Establish/maintain connections with client's significant people if client/community team have been unable to achieve this

Discharge

- Predict possible predischarge deterioration and wherever possible maintain the discharge day/hour in spite of deterioration
- Discharge may involve professionally appropriate risk (see "Professionally indicated risk-taking" section)

General principles of brief hospitalization *(cont.)*

Agreement/contract

♦ If there is agreement between client and staff that certain behaviours must stop, then:
  (a) Alternative options for behaviours must be given/explored/taught
  (b) Assistance given to develop these skills
  (c) Where possible, expectations that behaviour will decrease rather than stop immediately
  (d) Reinforcers drawn in to the contract

Client-controlled brief acute admissions

> I found the brief planned admissions useful for regrouping, although I did not use many. Four days was adequate for me and having a set of goals to achieve during the admission helped me to use them positively.
>
> (Jackson 1999)

Clients controlling their brief acute admissions could lead to large gains being made in current systems. Unfortunately, very little research has been done nor much written about this dimension of treatment. However, the principle is endorsed by a number of international experts. Nehls (1994) reported on a trial of five clients who essentially were in charge of their brief (48–72 hours) acute hospital admission rights. Results showed a 47% decrease in the number of days in hospital (25.8–13.8/client for the year). Some acute inpatient units have been using this system routinely with known clients for over a decade, where client and clinician collaboratively negotiate the duration, frequency and pathway for admissions and the contingencies around some behaviours.

The clinician will only contract with the client when the treating system is always able to meet their side of the contract, to admit the client when requested. To get around the unpredictability of a bed being available, one unit advises the client that if a bed is

not available, they will be able to attend the ward from 7 am.–
10 pm., with additional support offered if necessary overnight.
Another strategy is to indicate to the client an increased likelihood
of a bed being available on a weekend when some inpatients are
on weekend leave.

If the client is at sufficient acute risk of suicide, at the end of the
allotted time of the brief admission, they can stay in hospital.
However, the client-controlled brief, acute, admission contract
becomes null and void, with a return to traditional clinician-
controlled acute admissions.

The authors have had involvement with client-controlled brief
acute admissions for over 15 years and have heard over 100
anecdotal reports where this system has been used with positive
effect for client and clinician. Apart from Nehls' (1994) small
study, there is anecdotal literature (Geller 1993; Little and Stephens
1999) on the efficacy of such systems, but research is required.
Such research, if confirming the positive outcomes anecdotally
reported, would have far-reaching clinical impact.

Principles of the system are empowering of clients to be in
charge of their treatment, avoiding unnecessary power struggles
(which invariably the clinician can't win) and brief hospitalization
as a form of intensive respite and time out, but not a place of
"treatment". The communication to the client is, firstly, that acute
inpatient wards are usually a destructive place to be unless the
stay is brief, and secondly, that "treatment" takes place in the
community, not the acute ward. Such a system can take a huge
pressure off inpatient staff to "fix" the unfixable, leaving them
with the more manageable task of being warm to, rather than
trying to "treat" the client. The task is to reinforce, wherever
possible, the advantages of community-based treatment. Inpatient
clinicians are neutral and courteous but refer most matters to the
outpatient key clinician. This system can cut through the scenario
of clients exhibiting more and more extreme and dangerous
behaviour to demonstrate to clinicians the intensity of their
distress. The knowledge that admission remains a possibility can
have a "containing" effect, paradoxically preventing the need for
hospitalization.

Policies which could be considered on an individual basis include: a clear direction to staff to not build up intense individual relationships, having different staff each day attending to the client and having the outpatient key clinician and therapist see the client in their usual setting, not on the ward. These potential policies are controversial and have risks associated with them, especially that of dislocation and fragmentation of important healing relationships. Client-controlled, brief, acute admissions are dependent, for efficacy and efficiency, on a well-resourced outpatient treatment program that is "attractive" to the client.

A fictitious example of a client-controlled, acute admission contract

Agreement between A . . . and Goodenuf Mental Health Services

Summary

A . . . will be in charge of determining when she comes into hospital provided the conditions of the agreement are met by A . . . .

Whilst there will be exploration of the reasons for the admission, A . . . will not have to justify her admission.

In the event of the conditions not being able to be met by A . . ., then there will be a return to the situation where Goodenuf Mental Health Services determines whether A . . . is admitted to the acute inpatient unit.

Agreements

The pathway for A . . . to get into hospital is via IM Available (key worker) or IM Available's designated alternative

Maximum duration of hospitalization – 48 hours (or less at A . . .'s discretion)

Maximum number of hospitalizations – 2 per month. One at A . . .'s discretion and another if there has been no self-harm in the preceding 14 days.

Can only be admitted under this contract if no self-harm in previous 24 hours   yes/no

A fictitious example of a client-controlled, acute admission contract *(cont.)*

Can only be admitted under this contract if no illegal drug use in
previous 24 hours   yes/no

When admitted – continue outpatient clinical plan (No changes
to medication, therapy etc. This is the responsibility of outpatient team)

Overall key clinician/therapist seeing client during hospitalization yes/no

Participation in usual activities

Other contracts

(including contingencies, if any, for suicidal/homicidal statements
or self-harm)

The same principles of clients being in control of mental health
resources available to them have been applied to respite care when
systems have this capacity.

Pragmatic conceptual frameworks guiding treatment

Introduction

Clinically meaningful conceptual frameworks provide an important
foundation and guide to decision-making.

> Borderline patients require a flexible approach, and often put their
> therapists into a position of having to make instantaneous decisions in
> the middle of intense affect involving both patient and therapist.
> Without a current formulation which also includes the therapist
> monitoring of counter transference feelings, the needed therapist
> flexibility can easily be lost.
>
> (Adler 1993)

The conceptual frameworks of responsibility, clinician activity,
power, acute vs chronic suicide risk, short-term vs long-term gain/
risk and integration interweave with one another.

Responsibility

How much is the client and clinician responsible for in treatment and what is each party responsible for? Mary Graham (personal communication 1998), previous Executive Director and co-founder of the consumer-driven treatment organization S.A.F.E. in Canada (Self-Abuse Finally Ends), writes,

> As an ex-consumer who now works with consumers, I believe that each person should be held responsible for their own behaviours. The professional should work with utmost honesty and do whatever they can to help, but they should not be responsible for the client's behaviours. When a professional takes responsibility for their client's behaviour, they then develop a power struggle, which they will not win.

The issue of responsibility is a major recurring exploration point of treatment. Once the issue is adequately resolved, treatment has passed a significant watershed and client and clinician can more easily work collaboratively together.

> I had read books and I had heard 50 million therapists say that I was the only one who could make myself happy. I finally understood. If I didn't like what was going on, I could change it. No one else was going to do it. Being responsible for myself is power.
>
> (Everett and Nelson 1992)

> I really wanted someone to cure me and was irritated, to say the least, when it was suggested that I might, at least in part, be that someone. It took a long while and considerable conflict with mental health services to realize that the answer lay within myself. With the wonderful benefit of hindsight, I now see that eventually coming to this realization was a major turning point in my treatment.
>
> (Jackson 1999)

The reader will have met clients who, when asked how they might resolve their difficulties, state "You are the clinician, you tell me what to do". Such a response, whilst perfectly reasonable and understandable, is short of the ideal base for change to occur. From this position, which can be frustrating for both client and clinician, the task is to explore what the client and clinician are and are not capable of. This is often critical to change occurring.

Exploration of the advantages and disadvantages of self-sufficiency is pertinent. Positive aspects of self-sufficiency include being in control, determining one's future and not having to rely for one's well-being on other people, who are not always available, can't meet the desire or are untrustworthy. On the other hand, self-sufficiency includes doing things by oneself which are stressful, making difficult decisions which may not work out and opening oneself to failing. Clients may have all-or-nothing thinking around responsibility and self-sufficiency, which requires exploration. Self-sufficient people can choose to get support and can choose to invite others to share responsibility. The key difference is that the self-sufficient person has the choice and people who have choices tend to be happier. Self-sufficiency also can be associated with increased intimacy, connection and safety in relationships as the person is again relating from a place of choice.

Engagement of the client and commitment to the idea of change is crucial to the notion of self-responsibility. There are several stages of engagement. The first one is a tenuous engagement where the client is often desperate but has not yet made a connection to the clinician or team and does not yet have hope that change can take place.

Clinicians who encourage clients to take as much responsibility for treatment as possible, promote client feelings of empowerment, self-sufficiency, autonomy and being in control of their lives. Clinician flexibility is crucial, as holding too rigidly to the ideology of self-responsibility will result in the clinician declining to take enough responsibility. When the client is unable to do so for themselves this can lead to a deteriorating, destructive but preventable spiral. The levels of responsibility required by the clinician will vary from client to client, with the same client from session to session and sometimes within a session. A client's skill to carry out an activity, needs to be assessed. How this skill level changes and is influenced by the context and emotional state of the client, also needs to be assessed. (A client may be able to respectfully assert themselves with person A but unable to do so with person B. A client may have been successful at a task yesterday but unable to do the task today, because of heightened, distressing affect). There are no clear guidelines to advise the clinician as to how much responsibility to take, but principles of effective treatments, experience, training and supervision will assist development of skills required.

The clinician is responsible for carrying out clinical practice at a reasonable standard of care however, ultimately, the client with a diagnosis of borderline personality disorder is responsible for their behaviour (excluding psychosis, and some other Axis I disorders such as mania). There are often huge forces brought to bear on clinicians to disregard this simple notion. Pressures may come from clients, client's relatives and friends, other professionals, managers, police, lawyers, politicians and the media. When, as clinicians, we attempt to be responsible for clients' behaviour, we undermine the very foundations of successful treatment.

Fictitious clinical vignette

You are aware that your client is not getting her full financial entitlements from the government welfare service. You advise her of this. She makes contact with the welfare service but still doesn't get her entitlement. The extra money would make a critical difference. You explore ways she could improve her role. She tries again without any success. She is now angry at having to go cap in hand like a beggar. She is angry with you that you have not advocated for her on this matter. She has enough on her plate and doesn't need this and the demeaning put-downs that go with it. She vigorously argues for you to advocate on her behalf.

Fictitious clinical vignette

Your client in the past has communicated her distress by taking overdoses. During a scheduled session she shares her feelings of distress related to her friend recently moving to another city. In order to cope with these potentially overwhelming feelings she assertively and respectfully requests to increase the frequency of her sessions. You consider the dilemma. She has asked directly and overtly in a manner, which is likely to be beneficial for future relationships. This needs to be acknowledged and encouraged. On the other hand, she has a situation like this most of the time and you are eager to not reinforce a pattern that is going to lessen her self-capacities.

Fictitious clinical vignette

At the second outpatient session with you, your client indicates she is very suicidal which results in her hospitalization for 48 hours. At the fifth outpatient session she again indicates she is very suicidal leading to another 48-hour admission. At the seventh outpatient session she again indicates she is very suicidal.

Clinician activity

The level of clinician activity, like that of responsibility, will be determined by what is in the best interest of the client. As with the issue of responsibility, the more active the client is in treatment, the more will self-sufficiency and autonomy develop. A skills training, psychoeducational or cognitive-behavioural approach implies that the clinician has information to offer and will be reasonably active. The principle of getting the right balance of activity nevertheless still applies. As the client becomes more skilled and knowledgeable about themselves, it is appropriate they become more active and the clinician less active in the treatment. The clinician will have the flexibility to adapt their level of input for each individual client and with each client, as circumstances require.

Power

It is important that clinicians avoid, wherever possible, getting into a "fight" with the client. When researching a client population defined by nurses as "difficult", Breeze and Repper (1998) found both clients and clinicians feeling powerless in relation to one another. "... despite their different roles both nurses and 'difficult' patients were aware of the struggle to gain or retain a notion of control". It is little wonder that significant difficulties arise with both parties desperately trying to experience a semblance of control. From this position, an action from either party is quite likely to be experienced as further disempowering by the other party. It is useful for the clinician to step back and reflect that what feels like "power over" behaviour is likely to be an attempt by the client to deal with feelings of powerlessness. Whatever the clinician can do to assist the client to feel empowered (provided this is consistent with effective treatment principles), will lessen behaviour which clinicians experience as "power over".

Efforts to maximize collaboration can occur around developing a clinical plan, note taking, treatment and review. The process of treatment and the clinician's role can be demystified through a thorough orientation to treatment principles. Clinicians need to have a readiness to say "yes" to client requests, provided these activities encourage client goals, are within clinician limits and decisions are based on evidence-based treatment principles. This will not only directly improve client well-being but also the interactional dynamics between client and clinicians. "Where nurses were perceived to demonstrate respect, time, skilled care and a willingness to give patients some control and choice in their care, feelings of anger were reduced" (Breeze and Repper 1998).

Acute vs chronic suicide risk

Most people meeting diagnostic criteria for severe forms of borderline personality disorder are chronically suicidal, super-imposed on which, from time to time, is acute suicidality. The distinction between acute and chronic suicide risk where possible is critical as treatment interventions are very different and often quite opposite. When the risk is acute, it is appropriate for the clinician to be more active and interventionistic, for as short a period as possible. Gutheil (1985), an international medicolegal expert, writes,

> The central issue in acute suicidal state is a matter of despair, guilt and a consequent, usually short lived emergency state that requires immediate intervention. In contrast, the chronic suicidal state represents a seriously disturbed yet consistent mode of relating to objects in the environment. In this condition the central issue is the assumption of responsibility by the patient for his or her own life and its fate. The requisite interventions are not, as in an acute state, directed towards shepherding patients through a short term crisis until the self destructive press has passed, by somatic or psycho therapeutic approaches.

In a chronic situation it is counter-therapeutic for the clinician to take too much responsibility. "Taking the 'no-therapy' therapy approach advocated by Dawson and MacMillan (1993) can be helpful in side-stepping the imperative that the clinician take responsibility for the client's welfare" (Milton and Banfai 1999). "No-therapy therapy" advises the client that the therapist will be a warm active listener but is unsure of being able to be helpful beyond that. The therapist will be available but will not take responsibility for the client. Documentation of the chronicity of the suicidality provides important medicolegal protection.

The situation of acute on chronic suicidality is a familiar one requiring relatively more intervention in the short-term. The level of intervention will relate to the likely outcome of the client' action – predictable death must be stopped.

Short-term vs long-term gain/risk

> I have learnt to access services by being at risk and you reinforce this if you over-respond. Focusing excessively on suicidality stopped me from focusing on the important things behind it and therefore prevented change.
>
> (Jackson 1999)

To statistically increase the likelihood of the client being alive in the long term, one might need to make decisions whereby there is an increased possibility of suicide in the short term. This concept is one with which the community, the health profession, and even some within the mental health and legal profession are not familiar. The concept runs contrary to most life-threatening disorders. Undergoing risky surgery, however, provides a comparable model, except the risks and benefits are more concrete. Gutheil (1985) writes,

> To put this in crude as possible terms, the evaluator's choice, largely by hindsight, appears to lie between two outcomes – a concrete dead body and the rather abstract notion of personal growth. No wonder the decision is so charged with anxiety.

The Crisis Recovery Service (undated), The Maudsley provides a service for individuals who self-harm. In their philosophy and protocols booklet they write,

> It follows from an approach which insists on individuals taking responsibility for their own behaviour that risks to the short-term safety of residents may need to be taken in the interests of their long-term safety and health.

Integration

Black and white, all-or-nothing and dichotomous thinking describe similar processes to intrapsychic splitting (see section "Staff differences"). The processes of moving to extremes and polarities occur in clients, clinicians and treating teams. The task for client, clinician and treating team is to integrate and synthesize their different parts. The pathways to integration may include as a base: recognition of the concept, recognition that there are parts of oneself or the team that are not integrated, a desire to change and a safe environment to consider less well thought of parts. On this base, other pathways include alertness to the process occurring, oneself or others identifying the possibility of the process occurring, reflection, feedback and practising alternatives.

Cognitive behavioural strategies

Work using behavioural chain analysis, cognitive inferences and core beliefs/schemas can be found in standard cognitive behavioural texts, as can information on impulse control, tension/distress reduction and self-soothing. However, it is probably best to use texts which are focused on people meeting diagnostic criteria for borderline personality disorder, because of the modifications required for this group (Beck *et al.* 1990; Layden, Newman, Freeman and Morse 1993; Linehan 1993a; Linehan 1993b; Young 1994). There are also many popular psychology books available for clients and relatives/friends using these principles.

DBT skills training is well manualized for clinicians with many handouts for clients. DBT skills training is divided into two areas: acceptance skills and change skills. The acceptance skills are mindfulness skills and distress tolerance skills. Mindfulness skills (including observing and describing behaviours, thoughts and feelings) develop capacity for concentration and focusing the mind on the task in hand. Observing and describing assists with self-reflection and provides important data for chain analysis. Observing distress can decrease impulsivity and invites the concept that distress can pass without action. Distress tolerance skills include "distraction, self-soothing, improving the moment and thinking of pros and cons" as well as accepting that which can't be changed nor improved upon (Linehan 1993b). The change skills are interpersonal effectiveness and emotion regulation skills such as knowing and acceptance of one's feelings and reducing vulnerability by tending to sleep and health needs. Further information can be found in the *Skills training manual for treating borderline personality disorder* which accompanies the text *Cognitive-behavioral treatment of borderline personality disorder* (Linehan 1993a; Linehan 1993b).

Cognitive behavioural methods of skill training and chain analysis have been used synergistically with Dawson's "no therapy therapy" approach. When used in this manner, the clinician is warm and constant and actively shares their knowledge. The clinician communicates that they have skills to share with the client and that they are neutral as to whether the client uses this skill and knowledge.

An outline of impulse control, distress reduction, self-soothing and mood modulating skills is in the tables below.

Impulse control skills

Definition

The skills to be able to choose to have a gap between an event and personal action

Strategies

- Valuing long-term goals
- Attempt to delay gratification
- Slow down thought processes/actions (a "long fuse"; a "Morris Minor" not a "Ferrari")
- Emotional observation, self-monitoring and behavioural chain analysis

Pathway

- Awareness of desire to action
- Name the possibility of impulsivity (if I do this, is there a possibility I will regret it?)
- Delay action whilst:
  Consider purpose of action
  Consider advantages and disadvantages of immediate action (especially short vs long term)
  Consider a range of possible immediate actions (including doing nothing)
  Choose the best action
- Carry out action

Distress reduction and self-soothing skills will be i
and client determined. The clinician can name some possi
but the client will probably know best what has and has not been
effective in the past. What is useful for one person might make
things worse for another.

Distress reduction skills

Decrease physiological arousal – (various relaxation techniques)

- Progressive muscle relaxation (tense and relax)
- Muscle relaxation (relax only)
- Breathing skills
- Posture (Laura Mitchell, Alexander technique, Yoga)
- Meditative (audiotape with words, music)
- Meditation – unstructured
- Meditation – structured

"Grounding" (especially useful for dissociation)

- Increase kinaesthetic sensations (feet on floor, back against chair)
- Increase auditory and visual sensations (look around, here I am)

Visual imagery especially if self-designed (well-being, safety, connection, spiritual)

Usual cognitive strategies for anxiety

(it will end, it's only anxiety, it's OK to be anxious, I have been here before and I did OK)

Behaviour/activity

- Pleasurable activities (sense of well-being)
- One thing at a time is effective
- Distraction, whilst avoidant, can break a deteriorating spiral. Common distractions: gardening, walking, sport, reading. "Better to kill time than to kill yourself" (Stone 1990b)

Distress reduction skills *(cont.)*

Acceptance of what can't be changed
- This involves not fighting the distress thereby making it worse

Transitional items
e.g. cuddly toy, blanket, item gifted by important person

Personal crisis plan
- List of what works, whom to contact etc. (Kept by client at all times)

Self-soothing skills

Cognitive (affirmations, self-talk) (especially safety, connection and affirmation of worth)
"My body is deserving of being looked after"
"People around me now are different from those who abused me"
"There are people who want to be with me"

Behavioural
Pleasurable activity e.g. bath, music etc.
Meaningful activity e.g. prayer
Creative activity (dance, paint, write, draw)
Successful activity (do something one is good at)

Visual imagery especially if self-designed (well-being, safety, connection, spiritual)
Create safe and soothing visual images to return to at will
Meet your own wise person, meet your own protector, retreat to your safe place
Metaphors (e.g. dragons to protect, blankets to nurture)
e.g cuddly toy, blanket, item gifted by important person

Self-soothing skills *(cont.)*

Place of safety

Place of retreat specially designed to meet unique needs

Transitional options

Mindfulness of pleasurable experiences

e.g. speaking to friend, showering, walking in the sunshine, helping friend, watching a movie

Mood modulating skills

Goal

Having the capacity to consciously turn up and down the intensity of one's feelings

Mood modulating skills include

Impulse control skills
Distress reduction skills
Self-soothing skills
Behavioural chain analysis
Awareness, labelling and acceptance of feelings
All our feelings are O.K. (behaviour may not be). However we only need small doses of guilt and shame
Disengaging from situations likely to be destructive
Nurturing physiological state (sleep, nutrition, tending to health)

Cognitive statements which clients have frequently found useful follow. (Clients generally resonate more with the term "self-talk" than cognitive statements). The strategy is to deliberately challenge and replace thoughts which are not helpful (e.g. I am totally useless) with constructive thoughts (e.g. I am skilful at . . .).

Cognitive statements: self-talk

"My body is deserving of nurturance and care"

"I can communicate effectively with words"

"I am able to cope with unpleasant feelings"

"I am like this because of what happened to me" (Externalising causality)

"Most people would have ended up similar to me, if they had the same experiences"

"I am doing the best that I know how (to survive)"

"I was powerless (a child) at the time and could not prevent the abuse"

"I was not responsible for the abuse"

"I am not a bad person because of the abuse"

"I did not deserve the abuse"

The table below lists physical, cognitive and behavioural possibilities which clients may find useful in dealing with flashbacks during the "stabilization" phase of treatment (see section "Prioritizing interventions"). During this phase the primary goal is to get out of the flashback experience without being overwhelmed.

Coping with flashbacks during stabilization phase of treatment

Self-talk

"This is a flashback – I am not crazy"

"I have been here before and got through it"

"I have been through hard times before"

"I didn't cause the abuse and am not a "bad" person because of the abuse"

Grounding
Self-talk

"These are flashbacks – they are not real in present time"

"The date on the calendar, which I can see is . . ."

"The time on my watch is . . ."

Coping with flashbacks during stabilization phase of treatment (cont.)

Physical

Tactile – Feel my back against chair, my feet on the ground, my breathing

Hearing – My name is ... It is ... (day/date). Speaking self-talk statements aloud

Sight – "I can see ... (familiar safe things)"

Smell – "I can smell ... (familiar safe smells)"

Taste – "I can taste ... (familiar safe tastes)"

Contact

Speak to safe familiar people

Self-soothing skills

Distress reduction skills

Personal hierarchy of written things to do when having flashbacks

Once stability has been achieved and trauma is being explored, a treatment goal may be to stay in the flashback deliberately despite distressing but not overwhelming feelings as a means of "working through" or "exposure" to the material. "Having flashbacks can be an important part of my healing".

Behaviour chain and solution analysis

A chain analysis starts with identification of the problem (e.g. cutting, overdosing) followed by a moment to moment analysis of behaviours, thoughts and feelings preceding the problem behaviour and immediately after the problem behaviour. This provides the data for the solution analysis (exploration of how the client could do things differently in the future). The following two fictitious clinical vignettes trace a client's thoughts, feelings and actions as they evolve through the therapy process. The process has been outlined in a simple, abbreviated, straightforward manner to highlight the pathway and desired impact over time, of behaviour chain and solution analysis. The situation is rarely as straightforward as described.

Behaviour chain and solution analysis – fictitious clinical vignette 1

> *Client:* I am so upset with her – she ought to know the pain I am in – she doesn't care about me – I can't stand it – I will phone her, I'm sure she will understand – She is not in – it's not fair – I feel like breaking the phone – I break the phone – Oh no! Now she can't return my call – I am so alone – nobody in the world cares about me – I am totally useless – I will take an overdose – then the pain will go away.

Comment: There is a cascade of triggering events, thoughts and feelings occurring at a furious pace, gathering increased momentum like an avalanche. The client appears to be exercising limited active choice and control of her feelings. Inferences are made without evidence (she ought to know the pain I am in; she doesn't care). There are some belief systems which are absolutist and likely to lead to further disappointment and distress (people ought to know the pain I am in; I can't stand it; if I phone her, she will understand; the world should be a fair place). Core schemas rapidly rise to dominate the situation (nobody cares about me; I am totally useless).

> *Client:* I am so upset with her – she doesn't understand me the way I would like – I am having doubts whether she cares about me – I am so distressed but I can stand it – I have felt this way before and got through – I will phone her – maybe she will understand – She is not in – Oh no! Now what am I going to do? – Last time I broke the phone and that made things worse – I feel so alone – I wish there was somebody around who could care for me – Jill said I could ring her when I felt down – If she is not in, I will just take an overdose.

Comment: The sequence of events is somewhat slower. The client is using self-talk (cognitive strategies) (I can stand it – I have felt this way before and got through it) and less black and white, absolutist thinking (she doesn't understand me *the way I would like*; I am distressed *but I can stand it*; *maybe* she will understand). The expectation that things should be a certain way just because she wants them to be, is no longer evident. This is likely to lead to less disappointment and will slow down the previously escalating cascade. After being unable to speak to the person, she delays action using impulse control skills (stop, think – what am I going to do now?), draws and learns from past experiences (breaking the phone made the situation worse) by weighing up the disadvantages and advantages of breaking the phone. She experiences feelings of aloneness but is able to stay with these feelings in a more accepting way rather than being enveloped by harsh, critical schemas of nobody caring about her and being useless. In fact, she recalls someone who said to ring at these times – a caring offer. By taking some action to deal with her aloneness (ring Jill) she has moved out of her previous passive position. The course of action may be effective and she could use this to dispute the previously activated schema that she was totally useless. However, her repertoire of alternative options to overdosing runs out if Jill is not available.

> *Client:* I am so upset with her, I feel so hurt – I would like to feel she understood me better – I am finding this difficult but my strategies for dealing with distress are helping – I will phone her – If I share my feelings with her, she may understand better. However, I will be ready, in the reasonable eventuality, that it makes no difference – She is not in – I am aware of feeling increasingly alone – I will look at my crisis plan because I know when I get this distressed, I don't think as clearly as I would like – My crisis plan, which I wrote, says to find safe people and places to be and to nurture myself – I will ring Jill and if she is not in, Gail – If Gail is not in, I will take a hot bath with bath salts, read my book by the fireplace and then go to sleep. I usually feel better the next day – Whilst I would prefer to be with someone, I can always be a good friend to myself. Gee – this therapy stuff may be of some use after all – a few months back I would have smashed things and ended up in hospital. Whilst I have had support, I have done it. Maybe I will have a life worth living after all.

Comment: She is using many more "I" statements, which imply she is taking control of the situation and things that she can change. She has identified and named feelings of hurt for the first time. This provides a focus for her to tend to in the future. Her thoughts and feelings are less black and white and absolutist and more integrated (she *may* understand better, however I will be ready in the reasonable eventuality that it makes no difference; whilst I would *prefer* to be with someone, I can always be a good friend to myself). She is sufficiently in control to remember her crisis plan and to get it and read it. She plans a crisis hierarchy (ring Jill, failing which ring Gail, failing which a bath, book and sleep). She is ready to nurture and self-soothe (bath, bath salts, book by the fire). These activities are also probably serving as distraction strategies. She is able to hold onto her distressing feelings without impulsive action at least till the next day (I usually feel better the next day). This statement enables her to think beyond the immediate moment and is accepting of the notion that she will have painful feelings, which will, in time, pass. She ends by an awareness of gains that she has made and reinforces herself. She feels empowered (I have done it) and there are glimmerings of hope for the future.

Behaviour chain and solution analysis – fictitious clinical vignette 2

> *Client*: He is late – How could he do this to me – I am so uptight – I am going to cut myself – I am cutting myself – I am feeling better. A normal person would not do this to themselves.

Comment: Whilst it may be accurate, an inference has been made without evidence that he could reasonably have been on time and that he has been inconsiderate. At this stage there is insufficient information to determine this – his car could have broken down. She is able to identify being "so uptight" but is unable to identify the feeling state beyond this. There is no consideration of alternatives to cutting, which appears to have occurred without a conscious decision to choose to cut. There is a rapid progression from realising he is late to cutting. Cutting is effective in dealing with the distressing feelings so she will continue to cut to deal with similar situations until she learns alternative skills. She ends by criticizing herself which is likely to create secondary feelings of shame, which will sustain her feelings of poor self-worth. The clinician's task is to assist development of further skills using a chain analysis, exploration of cognitive inferences and possibly schemas, distress reduction, mood modulation and self-soothing skills. Problems need to be identified and solutions explored.

Client: He is late – How could he do this to me? – I am so angry – I feel like a bomb about to explode – I hate him – I feel like cutting – The first step is to stop for a few seconds – Take 10 slow, deep breaths – How can I deal with my anger in other ways? – Now consider possibilities – Cutting, burn his sports magazines, dig in garden, eat a tub of ice cream – Digging sounds best – Dig vigorously in garden – I am feeling a bit better – still angry though – If I had cut myself it would have made sense, but digging in the garden is better for me.

Comment: The feeling of anger has now been identified and labelled which begins to enable the client to do something about it. Feeling like a bomb about to explode is not an unusual metaphor used by clients to describe emotions when action is imminent and can be used as a marker for the client to rapidly use pre-planned strategies. "I hate him" is likely to be a black and white response that lacks synthesis of the whole person. This will not enhance mood modulation (I love him – He is late – I hate him – and maybe in due course – I love him). After the automatic thought of cutting arises, she briefly delays action using impulse control (stop for a few seconds and 10 breaths) and distress reduction (10 slow deep breaths) skills – This enables identification of the problem – how am I going to deal with my anger constructively so that I don't make it worse for myself – She brainstorms a few possibilities, briefly considering advantages and disadvantages of each and proceeds to dig in the garden. She is still struggling with her anger, but is able to hold onto this without being overwhelmed. She praises herself for having not cut thereby increasing the chance of not cutting in the future.

Client: He is late – How could he do this to me – I am so angry – I must try deal with my anger in a way that doesn't make things worse – I have to learn to tolerate being angry – Whilst I am angry with him now, I know I also like him – I have written a crisis plan for these sorts of situations which is in my bag – Oh yes, my crisis plan says to not rise to assumptions without evidence and to give myself a treat (e.g. go to a street cafe) for not acting on impulse – I will go to a street cafe which will also distract me – I will wait to hear from him why he was late before I decide how to respond – I have done well – I have not overreacted. I have also been in control, accepted and looked after myself.

Comment: Skills are being further developed. Angry feelings are identified. She recognizes the potential for destructive behaviour and coaches herself towards a constructive outcome. Black and white thinking has been replaced with a synthesis of her whole feelings towards him and not dominated by the current moment. She is in sufficient control to recall that she wrote a crisis plan and to access and act on the plan. The concepts of impulse control, reinforcing herself (having a treat) for not being impulsive appear to be integrated into her thinking and she adds the concept of distraction. She defers any inferences from his lateness until she has more evidence. She finishes by affirming how well she has done, thereby increasing the likelihood of her trying this pathway again.

> *Client:* He is late – I hope he is OK – I wonder why that is – His car could have broken down or perhaps he is an unpunctual but nice person or perhaps he is an inconsiderate jerk – I won't know until I hear from him –– Oh well, no big deal – this gives me an opportunity to finish that book – Gosh I am getting better and better at this stuff and I have made it work for me.

Comment: Further skills have developed. The whole situation is calm and not intensely charged as before. She is feeling sufficiently OK to consider him (I hope he is OK). She uses Socratic, open-ended exploration of reasons for his lateness. She gets on with her life in a manner that is nurturing. She reinforces herself – naming her successes and her self-sufficiency.

Teams

Team structure

People meeting diagnostic criteria for borderline personality disorder have tended to receive treatment that is fragmented and reactive. Poor outcomes have then been used as evidence of the inefficacy of treatment. A cohesive team structure, essential for all areas of mental health, is even more critical in this area. When life and death decisions need to be made, staff differences will frequently be evident. A cohesive team structure, integrated services and clearly defined guidelines assist these differences to be constructive rather than destructive.

The key clinician role takes on even more importance in those clients with extreme and complex needs. The client often becomes objectified ('the client who does...') and this has serious dangers for client outcome. The system can become blaming of the client and each other, and is often unable to manage the hostility or fear created in the situation. What frequently occurs is that there are multiple agencies involved who all know the behaviours of the client, but there is no well held client history or formulation from the perspective of the client, to guide interventions. Keeping the client 'in mind' is often lost in desperate attempts to reactively manage the situation.

At the core of the team structure is the client and key clinician working wherever possible in collaboration. The key clinician, who may or may not be the therapist, is usually the clinician who has the most client contact and coordinates treatment with the client. The key clinician's roles usually include discussion of goals, contracting, education, safety assessment, developing and coordinating a clinical plan and monitoring progress. As outlined in the section on "Investing Value and Status in the Key Clinician Role", the key clinician needs to be trained, supported and empowered to lead and determine the clinical plan. The key clinician ensures that all relevant parties are involved in developing the clinical plan, wherever possible in agreement with it, know their role in the clinical plan and are consulted and informed of any changes made. Relevant parties within the treatment agency may include: outpatient, inpatient, crisis, respite, day program, prescribing clinician, substance use, emergency services, child and forensic services. Relevant external agencies may include: caregivers, family, private therapist, general practitioner, child protection services, police and lawyers (see table below). Roles and treatment goals need to be clear. A clear, transparent and coherent team structure minimizes fragmentation of treatment and assists the calm, considered following through of the clinical plan.

Team Structure

Internal to Treatment Organization

Inpatient Team	Crisis Team	Respite
Emergency Services	Day Program	Medication

Key Clinician

Client

External to Treatment Organization

Family/friends	General practitioner	Other treating
	Police	professionals
Other treatment		Child protection
organizations		agencies

Investing value and status in the key clinician role

> "The reward system should more adequately support those therapists who care for the patients often avoided by others"
>
> (Robbins, Beck, Mueller and Mizener 1988)

The key clinician, who may or may not be the therapist, and is usually the clinician who has the most client contact, coordinates treatment with the client. This role requires many multifaceted skills including establishing an alliance, developing a clinical plan, monitoring progress, communication and psychoeducation (Gunderson 2001). The key clinician needs to face personal, medicolegal and career risks and challenges (suicide of a client, complaints, media and public expectation) without undue anxiety. Life and death professional decisions need to be made for which guidelines are very limited. Frequently, the clinical situation requires these decisions to be made on the spot by the clinician alone, without involvement of others. The leadership qualities required are considerable. With multiple agencies involved, the key clinician needs to lead a "team" which is different for each client, where "team" changes occur frequently and where the team's only commonality is involvement with the client. As well as the capacity for autonomous functioning and holding of considerable responsibility, the key clinician needs to function well as a team person. The key clinician role is probably the most important role in the treatment of this group and needs to be invested with accordingly high value and status. Practical demonstrations of value and status could include training, supervision, ongoing educational opportunities, sufficient time dedicated to the work and a pay scale commensurate with the difficulty.

Specialist teams

Specialist teams may provide direct client treatment in outpatient, day, inpatient or residential settings or a combination of these settings. Staff who have interest, experience and training are gathered together to provide a service at a higher or specialist level for clients whose treatment has not been effective in treatment as usual contexts. Having motivated, experienced and trained staff who have a specific focus assists the development of an effective treatment culture maximizing principles of effective treatment. These specialist teams need to be well linked with generalist teams to ensure that generalist clinician skills in treating people meeting diagnostic criteria for borderline personality disorder are not lost but maintained or maximized. This can be done by training, sharing treatment and consultation.

Specialist consultation teams may provide primary, secondary or tertiary consultation. In primary consultation the consultant sees and assesses the client and offers an opinion around the appropriate treatment pathway. This may include diagnostic issues, medication, psychotherapy and other therapy options. The strength of this approach is having an authorative expert lead the way. A disadvantage is that frequently a treatment pathway needs to evolve over time and in the context of complex client–clinician and clinician–clinician relationships. Having a one off consultation may work reasonably well around diagnostic issues but may be too linear, overly simplistic or not be cognisant of the need for a treatment plan to develop over time and a number of meetings. Secondary consultation is mindful of these issues. In this model the team treating the client refers the case to the specialist who spends time with the treating team assisting them to establish a therapeutic treatment plan, and supporting the team to resolve their own dilemmas and conflicts about the treatment. The specialist consultant may or may not offer group supervision to the team, or they may act in a role which assists the team to take up the work in a confident manner. In a tertiary consultation model the specialist consultant works with the service delivery system to ensure better client outcomes. Here, the specialist consultant engages with management, policy makers and clinicians to maximize treatment options for the client group. This may involve training and staff development and the establishing of policies, procedures and guidelines.

Systems

Every client who has moderate to severe levels of difficulty with their lives has engagement with one or more systems of health care. The complexity of the issues and the multiple agencies all with differing philosophies, entry criteria and models of service delivery, can make for a potent mix for good for the client or a destructive and dangerous process, in spite of good intentions.

The systems can involve outpatient services, inpatient services, community, rehabilitation and housing agencies as well as a therapist, family and the justice system among others. In order to progress a clear, coherent and therapeutic plan, there are times when it is useful to have an outside consultant to assist staff to work through the complexities and ensure that any hostility or negative affect do not find their way into the clinical plan.

Responsiveness of the organization to clinician needs

People meeting diagnostic criteria for borderline personality disorder pose particular difficulties for the clinicians closest to them. Clinicians often feel overwhelmed and can react in counter-therapeutic ways in order to protect themselves. Clinicians require an interpersonal environment that can contain their anxiety. "A program, group or clinician cannot contain more anxiety than the system can" (Owen 1998). The clinician requires a "sufficiently resilient holding environment that apprehends the psychic pain of clients and can bear the pain of being unable to relieve the pain" (Owen 1998). In order for clinicians to constructively process and weather the client's fluctuating, intense behavioural and feeling states (including anger and devaluation), and keep a positive warm relationship with the client alive, the organization requires a number of structures to be in place. A clear, practical set of policies, procedures and guidelines need to be written and fully supported at all levels of the organization.

Senior staff need to be available for assisting with difficult decision-making, recognizing that decisions are often made in the midst of intense, highly charged crisis situations. Clinicians require active support around the results of decisions they make, within a context of reasonable standards and the staff member having a history of competent clinical practice. Satisfactory, reasonable decisions can result in negative outcomes, and senior staff need to support clinicians in both internal and external forums, such as the coroner's court. This means that any one person (especially junior staff) involved with a client does not bear the brunt of the organization having accepted an inherently risk-filled, but actively planned and sound treatment plan. Organizations and people assessing critical incidents need to recognize that decision-making in highly charged situations is much more difficult than at other times.

As the therapist's task is to be 'good-enough' for the client, so the organization's task is to be 'good-enough' for the clinician (Owen 1998). Dealing with conflict and difference is an essential task for the client, clinician and the organization. "The amount of conflict and difference a clinician can constructively process is directly related to the amount that the organization can process" (Owen 1998). At all levels of the organization, linkages can be fostered which protect both the clinician and the client, by providing a confident, calm, clear environment for staff to provide treatment.

In summary, key system features are:

◆ clear policies, procedures and guidelines
◆ focused coherent and skilled supervision

+ senior clinical staff and management support
+ a confident, calm, clear environment
+ a capacity to resolve conflict and difference

Staff differences

The term "splitting" originated out of the description of the phenomenology of clients being seen to "split" themselves, so to speak, into different parts, with each part dominant at any one time and with limited capacity to integrate the constituent parts into a cohesive whole. People are related to as part-people, rather than integrated whole people. People will be perceived as either all-gratifying or all-persecuting with associated idealization and devaluation. An example is adoring someone one moment followed by intense, all-encompassing hatred in response to a perceived slight. An example of integration is the capacity to feel angry feelings for someone that at the same time you know you like. Historically, staff members frequently found themselves identifying with a part-dimension of the client without integrating this into the whole dimension. Out of these experiences it was hypothesized that clients actively "split" staff.

Whilst these phenomena have been very important in assisting understandings of the rapidly fluctuating internal and external states of clients and the on/off relationships clients frequently have, the term "splitting" is now contaminated and polluted with inappropriate associations. For some clinicians, it may incorrectly imply deliberate malevolent intent of a client to create staff differences, rather than the client's best possible means of coping. The implication may be one of a "bad" client. Conflict occurs around many difficult clinical scenarios where there are intense feelings, difficult situations and high anxiety. The service is, in effect, being challenged in its capacity to process staff differences.

Probably the most significant risk in using the term "splitting" is that staff members believe something is being done to them, taking a passive, pessimistic victim position and thereby disempowering themselves. From this self-created, disempowered position, staff members disavow the obvious interactional dimension to the phenomena and do nothing to address the problem. Gunderson (2001) emphasizes the interactional nature of splitting and is quoted (Cauwels 1992),

> The danger in seeing splitting as too much of an intrapsychic problem and not enough of an interactive one is that it underestimates the capacity of clinicians and other people to correct it.

It is easy to see how this will lead to an escalation of bitterness, anger and resentment, which is so destructive for clients and staff alike. An alternative description of "staff differences" or "conflict" goes some way towards dealing with the problem. It is completely normal for human beings to have differences, especially around life and death issues. Using the term "staff differences" also makes it clear whose problem this is. If staff members have differences, it is the staff members' task to find a way through this. Whilst the client may have a contributory role, it is the staff's task to address solutions.

The greatest differences amongst staff members occur around how nurturing or limit-setting to be. Such differences are entirely normal and to be expected. An environment that encourages respectful expression of these differences will paradoxically decrease staff members moving to extreme positions. Staff members are more likely to feel seen, heard and understood (although not agreed with) and less likely to take a radical polar position in order to be seen and heard. In this manner the culture will assist integration and synthesis of part positions. A culture that does not enable individuals to feel heard is likely to encourage staff to polarizing positions and behaviours. Some staff members will identify with the client's traumatized past and current distress and wish to respond with compassion and caring. An understanding of this "victim" dimension of the client is accurate and true but only a part of the whole picture. Other staff members will identify with the verbal and other abuse of the client and wish to respond with firm limit-setting. An understanding of this "perpetrator" dimension of the client is again accurate and true and again is only a part of the whole picture. These polarized positions are no longer in the healthy difference domain and invoke terms such as "enmeshed, overinvolved, withholding and punitive". The synthesis, of polarized part-positions into a whole, is a central task for each clinician, for the treating team and for the client. The continuum in the table below emphasizes that differences are normal and to be expected. However, when individuals hold an extreme position, problems arise.

Staff differences

←――――――――――――――――――――――――――――――――――→

Enmeshed	Nurturing style	Limit-setting style	Withholding
Over involved (identification with "victim" dimension of client) (Unhealthy difference)	(healthy difference)	(healthy difference)	Punitive (identification with "perpetrator" dimension of client) (Unhealthy difference)

The task is for individuals and the treatment team to synthesize the part-perspectives of "victim" and "perpetrator".

In the synthesis, differences will remain but will now be in the healthy difference domain.

The task is to have a culture which encourages diversity, provided:

  the diversity is within ethical and medicolegal boundaries
  the team are not pulling in diametrically opposite directions
  the diversity is consistent with knowledge of effective treatment principles.

"It costs time and courage to learn how to sit in the fire of diversity. It means staying centred in the heat of trouble" (Ryan, 1997).

Principles of a team/system culture which will proactively assist the addressing of staff differences

Cohesion

Cohesion requires of individuals the capacity to let go of what we personally consider to be the best way in favour of a larger, more important perspective.

This perspective values cohesion and consensus above individuality, provided treatment is within effective treatment principles

Characteristics of an effective treatment network

Cohesion

Fluidity (adaptability to change)

Sub-teams linked to each other (inpatient, outpatient, crisis, substance use etc.)

Treatment network links to other networks (welfare and housing agencies, emergency department, police, child protection agency etc.)

Characteristics of strong communities

Encourage participation

Flexible

Manage diversity

Good leadership

Regulate behaviour through formal and informal rules

Consequences are more often natural than arbitrary

Constituted parts are balanced

People have a sense of belonging

People are positively integrated with the community

People are interdependent

Adapted from and reprinted with permission – Gleisner S – personal communication, 1997

The following clinical vignettes are examples of scenarios of staff conflict or scenarios that *could* lead to staff conflict. They provide an opportunity to reflect on how to minimize the potential for polarization and how to explore and negotiate differences.

Fictitious clinical vignette

Client 1: I have something I would like to share with you, but am concerned that you might overreact.

Client 2: I have something I would like to share with you, but want it to remain just between the two of us. It has nothing to do with myself or anyone else being at risk, but it would help me if you knew this information.

Client 3: I have built up some trust in you and want to share something with you about my past. I don't mind others in the team knowing some of the outline of what happened but I don't want them to know all the details, as it is very private.

Fictitious clinical vignette

The client you have been seeing weekly in the community takes an overdose and is admitted to the acute psychiatric unit. There is ongoing communication between you and the unit staff with considerable professional conflict. Unit staff feel there is no evidence to support her history of being raped three times over the last year which leads them to wonder about the validity of her history of childhood sexual abuse. She has a one-month stay at the end of which she is discharged with a diagnosis of a factitious disorder.

Fictitious clinical vignette

Your client seeks out another clinician who thinks you are a kindly person but are preventing her capacity for independence and growth by encouraging her to be dependent on you. She has been seeing you weekly for seven months and both of you for the last eight weeks. She has seen the other clinician on three occasions at irregular intervals. You make contact with the other clinician and discuss your different views. The other clinician agrees to advise when further contact occurs. This doesn't happen.

Fictitious clinical vignette

Clinician 1 is the inpatient clinician responsible for admissions to the acute psychiatric unit. The unit is usually full with sub-optimal treatment because of insufficient staff. A client meeting diagnostic criteria for borderline personality disorder has had five one-week admissions in the last 15 weeks. Her admissions are because the community clinician felt she was suicidal. Whilst you recognize that the client could kill herself, you are less convinced that the hospitalizations in the long run are going to decrease the risk. In fact you are concerned that the hospital is in fact reinforcing her to remain unwell.

Clinician 2 is the community clinician. You believe that without the recent series of hospitalizations, the client would probably be dead. Because of the suicide risk, you are less concerned about dependency on the hospital, which can be attended to when the suicide risk is lower.

Residential treatment

Some clinicians advocate for a residential service for treating people meeting diagnostic criteria for the more severe forms of the disorder, using a model similar to the Cassel in England. The argument is based on the idea that severity should be matched with intensity. Most current clinical interest, academic interest and ongoing research is in community based models and to a lesser degree day programs. Undoubtedly some clients would respond better to residential treatment than to outpatient treatment. In an ideal situation, there would be a wide range of options to select from, enabling people to get treatment that would best suit them. Because of fiscal restraint, service delivery options in the public sector need to be made on the basis of what is in the public good. How are most people going to benefit from monies spent? Current evidence points strongly towards outpatient treatment being developed first.

The model of residential treatment provides for an intervention for a period of time and this can be a very important 'circuit breaker', However what is required for many of these clients is a longer term model. The authors experience is that for many people in residential treatment the quality of the outcome is dependant on the quality of the pre and post ongoing commitment of the treatment team. The good work of a residential program can be laid to waste if the treating team in the community is unavailable afterwards, or poorly developed. There is some empirical support for this in a preliminary report on treatment at The Cassel, a residential treatment facility. Whilst both groups improved, clients treated with six months residential treatment followed by community outreach and group psychotherapy did better than those receiving residential treatment (11–16 months) only (Chiesa and Fonagy 2000).

Financing a residential treatment facility before satisfactory outpatient services have been developed has six major disadvantages. Firstly, it deprives outpatient services of the resources required for effective treatment. Secondly, it encourages client and clinician to not give it their "best shot" with outpatient treatment because there is the "expert" residential service "out there" to whom a referral will be made. Thirdly, the ambience of "experts out there" encourages an "out of sight, out of mind, not our responsibility" culture. The workforce already sometimes avoids treating this group and needs no further system encouragement. Fourthly, the workforce outside the "expert" residential facility is where the vast majority of treatment will take place. A residential service may deskill the very staff who are doing most of the work. Fifthly, it would dislocate treatment when residential treatment was completed and the person moved on to outpatient treatment. People meeting diagnostic criteria for borderline personality disorder respond poorly to dislocations of important relationships. Lastly, if the population were scattered, centralizing a residential service would disadvantage people in other areas.

Residential services should be developed after the establishment of comprehensive outpatient services and with considerable thought and planning. To avoid some of the above problems, entry to the residential service could require each referring system to be satisfactorily resourced with finances, time and clinical skills and the referred client to have already had well-supported, proactively planned outpatient treatment over a significant time period.

Residential treatment can be potent, however caution needs to be applied to the type of person who can benefit and the resourcing of treatment for the most extreme and complex of needs. For some of these people a residential situation is too intense and the violence and more sadistic forms of self-harm are damaging to the other clients in the residential community. These individuals may be provided with better and more appropriate care in individualized programs in the community with appropriate supports and skilled case management.

Relatives and friends

> Learn all you can about the disorder; be realistic about how much
> support you can offer – this makes you more likely to stick around for
> the long haul; set limits and stick to them; don't fall into the trap of
> taking control.
>
> (Jackson 1999; A client's recommendations to relatives and friends.)

There is a paucity of literature and experience to guide clinicians in
this area, as historically most interest has been in direct work with
the client. This is appropriately beginning to change as clinicians
are exploring ways of constructive engagement with relatives and
friends. Relatives and friends live in a stressful environment and
have needs for assistance of their own. The problems and issues
that relatives and friends struggle with are, not surprisingly, similar
to those of clinicians.

Meeting with relatives and friends at the beginning of treatment
can often decrease the potential for destructive triangular
relationships and increases the likelihood of joining to enhance
treatment goals. Orientating relatives/friends to treatment and
prognosis can be helpful. Realistic expectations of what can and
can't be provided are discussed as well as a realistic time frame, if
recovery is to take place. Relatives and friends usually are aware
that there is a risk of suicide although have not always articulated
this. Introducing concepts of acute versus chronic suicidality and
short-term versus long-term risks/gains can assist relatives/friends
to support treatment strategies and provide the clinician with some
medicolegal protection.

A number of centres are exploring provision of psychoeducational and skills training groups which clients and relatives/friends
attend (Gunderson 1997; Gunderson 2001; Hoffman 1997).
Clients and families may have skill deficits that maintain the
disorder by each party reinforcing maladaptive behaviour. A
major goal of treatment is to assist clients and families together
acquiring skills to interrupt this cycle (Hoffman 1997). Concepts
may be shared of the client having skill deficits around emotion
regulation, impulsivity and difficulties feeling alone. Dichotomous,
all-or-nothing thinking and the need to synthesize polarities may

also be discussed. As these issues are on a continuum, relatives/ friends and clinicians are assumed to also be able to improve their skills in these areas. The focus is future orientated with clients and relatives/friends asked to consider how they could best contribute to improving the situation. Skills training occurs in areas of impulse control, affect regulation, distress reduction, self-soothing, assertion, social skills and conflict resolution.

Whilst clients are identified as having skill deficits, it is clear that they are responsible for their behaviour and for change. Relatives/friends are encouraged to be supportive, using principles consistent with effective evidence-based treatments such as trying not to be responsible for the client's behaviour. The concepts of clinical plans, crisis plans and crisis hierarchies are discussed. Relatives and friends are encouraged to also look after themselves and to sustain a life outside of that with the client.

Most clients have a significant person/s in the community interested in their well-being whom they may wish to have involved. However where relatives/friends are generally unsupportive of the client, or are abusing the client, clinicians need to be mindful of the possibility that less contact may be more beneficial than more contact, at least initially.

Clinicians may wish to read the booklets *The Self-Harm Help Book* (Arnold and Magill 1998) and *Working with Self-Injury* (Arnold and Magill 1996), a journal co-edited by a relative of an affected individual on borderline personality disorder *(Journal of the California Alliance for the Mentally Ill 1997; 8(1))*, the book *Stop Walking on Eggshells* (Mason and Kreger 1998), contact TARA APD (Treatment and Research Advancements Association for Personality Disorder, 23 Greene Street, NY, NY 10013, USA) who provide assistance for relatives/friends and look at the Bristol Crisis Service for Women Website *(http://www.geocities.com/Wellesley/)* to see whether they would consider any of these suitable to mention to client's relatives/ friends.

Principles of effective treatment

A summary of principles of effective treatment follows:

Principles of effective treatment

- Clients are responsible for their behaviour (excluding psychosis and some other Axis I diagnoses such as mania)
- A proactive clinical plan developed collaboratively between client and key clinician embodies integrated services (e.g. inpatient, outpatient, crisis, drug and alcohol)
- Intensive, proactive, structured treatment is available on an outpatient basis
- The clinician/system makes a long-term commitment to the client
- The client–clinician relationship serves as the foundation for effective treatment
- Acute hospitalization is avoided where possible by use of resourced alternatives
- Acute hospitalization when unavoidable is brief
- Acute hospitalization can only be avoided or brief when intensive community treatment exists
- Lengthy hospitalization (weeks) in acute psychiatric units is not encouraged and subject to routine local peer review
- Medication, if used, is an adjunct only to psychosocial treatments
- Mental health legislation is minimally used and when used is subject to local peer review (see "Clinical appropriateness of the use of mental health legislation" section)
- Supervision of significant involved clinicians is an essential part of treatment packages
- Clinicians feel supported by the institution/system
- The culture of the system is as important as the culture between clinician and client
- The effectiveness of the system is as important as the effectiveness of the clinician

In summary

- General and risk assessment is highly individualized
- A detailed history of past and current suicidality and self-harm will provide benchmark information required to develop a longitudinal treatment plan and to guide crisis treatments
- An identified key clinician is at the core of the team
- The key clinician role is probably the most important staff role in the treatment and needs to be invested with accordingly high value and status
- Key clinicians need to be empowered to determine treatment
- The client–clinician relationship provides the foundation for effective treatment
- A clinical plan created by client and key clinician is at the core of treatment
- Contracts are important
- "Whether a contract serves as a helpful adjunct to treatment or as a counter therapeutic distancing device, depends on how it is conceptualized, designed and negotiated" (McMahon and Milton 1999)
- The team culture ideally matters to the people who are part of it, is co-operative and mutually supportive and validates the clients, the work and the clinicians doing the work
- Key features of local systems are: clear policies, procedures and guidelines; focused, coherent and skilled supervision; senior clinical staff and management support; a confident, calm, clear environment and a capacity to resolve conflict and difference
- A long-term perspective (years) needs to be held
- Initial treatment is prioritized to that which will achieve greatest client stability
- Clients are responsible for their behaviour (excluding psychosis and some other Axis I diagnoses), not the clinician
- Clinicians are responsible for their professional behaviour
- Avoid a "fight" with the client, wherever possible
- Interventions for chronic suicidality are different from those for acute suicidality

- A careful, individualized, professionally considered, risk–benefit analysis, with a well-known client, in the context of current professional research and clinical thinking, may lead to a short-term risk being taken to enable the possibility of long-term gains
- The client, clinician and treating team's task is to integrate all-or-nothing, black and white, dichotomous, part object, splitting types of thinking, feeling and behaviour
- The goal of crisis work is to assist the client's return to their pre-crisis level of function and includes a hierarchy of actions which may include anti-suicide interventions
- Acute hospitalization is avoided, where possible, by use of resourced alternatives
- Acute inpatient stays are, wherever possible, brief (up to 72 hours)
- Keeping acute admissions brief requires clear understandings of the issues of acute versus chronic suicidality, short versus long-term risk and organizational support for professionally indicated risk-taking
- Brief, acute admissions are dependent for efficacy and efficiency on a well-resourced outpatient treatment program which is "attractive" to the client
- Client-controlled, brief, acute hospitalization holds considerable promise
- Cognitive-behavioural strategies include behavioural chain analysis, disputation of cognitive inferences and schemas, impulse, distress reduction and self-soothing skills
- Distinguishing self-harm intended to suicide from that intended for other reasons will critically influence treatment pathways
- Self-harm not intended for suicide is to relieve internal distress or for communication
- The commonest reason for self-harm is relief of internal emotional distress especially anxiety and anger
- Distinguishing the reasons for self-harm will critically influence treatment directions

- Treatment may involve a behavioural chain analysis of the sequence of events leading to self-harm, with the intention of the client becoming more aware of possible points to intervene differently in the future
- A harm-reduction model encourages the person, if they are going to self-harm, to do so in a manner less likely to be life-threatening, disfiguring, or causing permanent damage
- Orientating relatives/friends to the disorder, treatment and prognosis can be helpful
- Psychoeducational and skills training groups for clients and relatives/friends are being explored
- There is a place for specialist treatment teams. These teams need to address ways of maintaining and maximizing skills in generalist teams
- There are many inherent dangers in setting up "expert" residential treatments prior to establishing effective comprehensive community services
- Residential services can compliment existing effective comprehensive community services

Part 3

Stigma, language, clinician feelings, and resourcing

When people meeting diagnostic criteria for borderline personality disorder are valued, they will be seen as having a legitimate clinical condition (with proven treatment methods) and will have an opportunity to receive effective, appropriate treatment.

Stigma and discrimination

Unlike the stigma the community puts on mental illness, the stigma associated with borderline personality disorder has been shown to come from within the mental health profession (Fraser and Gallop 1993; Gallop, Lancee and Garfinkel 1989; Lewis and Appleby 1988). Sometimes there is individual and institutional avoidance of treating people meeting diagnostic criteria for borderline personality disorder. When they are seen, it may be with ambivalence or annoyance. Linehan (1995) describes how clients who come to services with a diagnosis of borderline personality disorder may already be disliked before they have even been seen.

Clients in treatment are often embroiled in clinician attitudes that are derogatory or deny the legitimacy of their right to access resources. Studies have demonstrated that clinicians have less empathy for people meeting diagnostic criteria for borderline personality disorder than other diagnostic groups and make more belittling comments (Fraser and Gallop 1993; Gallop, Lancee and Garfinkel 1989). Consumers have identified this stigma (Haswell and Graham 1996; Mazelis 1997; Mazelis 1998) and drawn parallels with the stigma associated with AIDS in the early 1980s (Mazelis 1998).

Some of the stigma may be linked to the impact on mental health professionals of having clients who do not tend to get better in the short term and also infringe the code of behaviour of the sick role: co-operation, appreciation, gratefulness. Lewis and Appleby (1988) argue that psychiatrists view people with "mental illness" as deserving of compassion because they have not caused their problems. People with personality disorder on the other hand are viewed as not having a "mental illness", seen as being in control of their behaviour and consequently not deserving of compassion. Consumers have commented similarly,

> Current politics are espousing the 'biology of mental illness' and therefore appealing for public compassion for the 'victims of disease'.

> Empathy is sought for victims of illness rather than survivors of horrors.
>
> (Mazelis 1998)

Epstein (Krawitz and Watson 1999), consumer consultant on numerous national committees, writes,

> One of the most healing things I have been able to do for myself has been to access my psych files through freedom of information legislation. I use a line when speaking to various groups, it goes like this: 'You know all the awful things you thought they were writing about you — they were'. People usually laugh, especially other consumers who can relate immediately to what I am saying about power. When I accessed my records, I discovered that the language used to describe me by mental health workers underwent a palpable change (for the worse) subsequent to my being diagnosed with borderline and other personality disorders. While undergoing treatment, I had experienced a discrepancy between denigrating attitudes and caring rhetoric as being a consequence (or symptom) of my own evil. It seemed that a personality disorder diagnosis was telling me that my whole being was wrong: that there was a fundamental inadequacy about me as a human person.
>
> (Reprinted with permission of the Mental Health Commission)

Language – negative terminology

Words are important carriers of information and significantly shape the future. Some commonly used terminology such as "PD", "worried well" and "just behavioural" delegitimizes clients, is offensive and almost certainly leads to poorer outcome. We need to explore terminology that is more helpful. "Attention seeking" might be better replaced with "in need of attention", "manipulation" with "manoeuvre", "worried well" with "walking wounded" and "greedy" with "in need". The term "splitting", as described earlier, whilst conveying an important concept, has frequently been corrupted to blame the client for all staff differences and depower clinicians to do anything about the situation. Therapists who hold non-pejorative conceptualizations of their clients have been shown to achieve better results as measured by a decrease in client self-harm episodes and suicidal thoughts (Shearin and Linehan 1992).

Clinician values and feelings*

"Clinician values significantly impact on service provided. Success of treatment is partly dependent on clinicians coping with their own feelings in reaction to the client. People meeting diagnostic criteria for borderline personality disorder do not fit into psychiatric services very well. These services generally deal with either: (a) psychotic patients whose distress is not easy to empathize with, and for whom clinicians are happy to take responsibility, or (b) clients with other Axis I diagnoses who are insightful, cooperative, and respectful. People meeting diagnostic criteria for borderline personality disorder are difficult to understand, often disagree with clinicians' advice, and lead to great staff suffering. The residual meaning of the term 'Borderline' may be that these clients are between services.

Descriptive systems like DSM-IV give an illusion of understanding, as they do not really illuminate aetiology or process. There is also an implied precedence of Axis I over Axis II, with some services being restricted to "proper" patients with Axis I diagnoses. The comorbidity of borderline personality disorder with substance disorder, eating disorder, psychoses and most of all with affective disorder is great and accurate formulation often difficult. Certainly descriptive and diagnostic skills are important in assessment. But prolonged searching for a diagnosis other than borderline personality disorder can be destructive. It must be possible to make a positive diagnosis of borderline personality disorder, not only by ruling out other diagnoses. And it must be possible to acknowledge the primary, long-term importance of borderline personality disorder even when criteria for major depressive episode or other Axis I disorders are met.

. . . .

*This section on clinician values and feelings was written by Dr. Nick Argyle, Clinical Director, Auckland Healthcare, Director, Balance program (borderline personality disorder treatment program), Auckland Healthcare, and Honorary Senior Lecturer, Department of Psychiatry and Behavioral Sciences, Auckland University (Krawitz and Watson 1999). Reprinted with the permission of the Mental Health Commission.

Clinicians may be praised by other staff for protecting them, by discharging or refusing access to people meeting diagnostic criteria for borderline personality disorder. This may be an easier goal than making the patient better. The negative feelings to a client can be felt by all members of a team or unit, so inappropriate action by individual staff is not so evident to the others. Faced by a client who is causing staff to suffer, who is challenging to the clinician because he/she does not understand them, and who they do not know how to best help, it is easy to either designate them as non-patients and exclude them from care, or be punitive and detain in hospital in a restrictive manner. This rejection or punishment counter-therapeutically reinforces for the client that the world is in fact punishing and/or rejecting. It is also reflected in the way mental health services are contracted for and individual units' entry criteria set. Often borderline personality disorder does not fit anywhere.

Medication does have a role in therapy, especially with comorbid problems, but drugs may be over-used. Medication can be a powerful distracter. Changing medication to deal with frequent crises and mood changes can dissuade the client and other staff from recognizing the importance of psychosocial interventions, or undermine ongoing psychological therapy. Of course, medication can be helpfully prescribed in conjunction with other therapy, but this needs to be done sensitively.

The application of mental health legislation is an all or nothing decision and this can mesh nicely with sudden swings in clinician feelings, for example from caring and understanding to anger and rejection. For a doctor, being legally responsible for someone you cannot understand is difficult.

As people meeting diagnostic criteria for borderline personality disorder take their toll on us and are hard to help with our traditional methods, we often distance ourselves from these clients and consider their problems as illegitimate or self-inflicted. Our desire to keep ourselves unscathed is one of the roots of the attitude in mental health culture that invalidates the problems of these clients. Financial resourcing of treatment is almost certain to be strongly influenced by such attitudes".

Resourcing

The history of the "untreatability" of people meeting diagnostic criteria for borderline personality disorder came out of the experiences of psychoanalysts who found this client group did not respond well to usual psychoanalytic treatments of the day and in fact frequently got worse. Consistent with knowledge at the time, this group was considered unsuitable for treatment. Cognitive behaviour therapists, with their focus on specific treatment targets and goals, were developing their treatments elsewhere and did not explore the treatment of this group. A few decades later both psychodynamic and cognitive behavioural clinicians began modifying their approaches and engagement with people meeting diagnostic criteria for borderline personality disorder. Out of this fresh engagement, positive research studies and publications have arisen. The belief that treatment was ineffective was understandable in the absence of outcome studies demonstrating efficacy. This history still contributes to the current reactive ad hoc and "haphazard" delivery of treatment (Clarke, Hafner and Holme 1995).

Often public mental health services respond to people meeting diagnostic criteria for borderline personality disorder only when they are suicidal. This encourages the very behaviours clinicians are trying to decrease. The need to develop services that will indicate to clients that their morbidity will be responded to without them having to be suicidal is clinically self-evident. In targeting those with the greatest severity, there is a danger of encouraging clients who fall below the threshold required for intensive treatment to exhibit greater pathology in order to access treatment. Increased funding will not solve the problem, but will shift the threshold and move the problem to less crucial client behaviours. This iatrogenic system problem requires further exploration.

The high suicide rate (10–36%) and high morbidity, combined with knowledge of effective evidence-based treatments, provides a solid argument for financial resourcing to be on a par with other conditions with similar mortality, morbidity and efficacy of treatment. For the most disabled group, the financial cost of well-considered, skilled, proactive treatment may not be much different from the financial costs of a reactive service, due primarily to the cost savings of decreased hospitalization (also decreased crisis and medical interventions) (see sections "Health resource usage" and "Health resource use after effective treatment"). The notion that clients are choosing to lead lives of misery when they could do otherwise, or that they are not trying hard enough, is fanciful in the extreme and indicative of the stigma that exists. This stigma needs to be named, discussed and challenged.

In summary

- There has been a stigma towards people meeting diagnostic criteria for borderline personality disorder within the mental health profession
- Negative or offensive language impacts on client outcomes
- Clinician values and feelings are critical determinants for effective treatment
- Stigmatization has led to discrimination, most evident in the paucity of intensive, proactive treatment for those most severely affected
- Often public mental health services only respond to this client group when they are suicidal. This encourages the very behaviours clinicians are trying to decrease
- The high suicide rate (10–36%) and high morbidity, combined with knowledge of effective evidence-based treatments, provide a solid argument for resourcing to be on a par with other conditions with similar mortality, morbidity and efficacy of treatment
- For the most disabled group, the financial cost of well-considered, skilled, proactive treatment may not be much different from financial costs of a reactive service, due to the cost savings of decreased hospitalization

Part 4

The legal environment

Medicolegal framework

Good medico-legal practice is synonymous with good clinical practice.

> We are asked to take someone who has been hurt in the context of an interpersonal relationship and to treat them in, of all things, an interpersonal relationship. The client has been injured in the very channel in which psychotherapy subsequently occurs. It is not going to be smooth going.
>
> (Briere 1995)

People meeting diagnostic criteria for borderline personality disorder represent a significant risk for clinicians and organizations providing service, particularly because of the possibility of suicide and complaints. Involvement of the media and other influential community people such as Members of Parliament increases this risk. Gutheil (1985) in the article "The medicolegal pitfalls in the treatment of borderline patients" explains how a lack of understanding about optimal treatment choices and risks involved may lead to clinicians being blamed for ineffective treatment even when that treatment is of a satisfactory or better standard. In the event of an undesirable outcome, clinicians need to demonstrate that they practised according to a "reasonable practitioner standard", not that they practised perfectly.

The clinical practice around individuals who self-harm or indicate suicidal intent or attempts on a frequent basis can be very difficult to manage. The balance between clinician responsibility and client responsibility is a finely tuned one. Whilst general guidelines are available, such guidelines unfortunately are unable to specifically advise what to do in each unique crisis situation. Mental health has poor support from the community in terms of suicide. There is less distress and blame when someone dies from a medical or surgical disorder than when an individual suicides. There is often a tension between the fear of litigation and the desire to practice effectively. If there is a culture of fear of litigation then overly defensive practices inevitably occur associated with poorer outcomes.

Duty of care and institutional responsibilities

When a clinician sees a client a "duty of care" is owed by the individual health professional to the client. This means that the assessment and treatment by the health professional must be clinically sound and of a "reasonable practitioner standard". A duty is also owed by the health institution, which is non-delegable. This means the employer has a duty to ensure an appropriate infrastructure exists to enable effective clinical standards to be met. In many countries the institution bears a liability for ensuring good practice occurs. This is evidenced in training programs around managing high-risk clients, training in assessment procedures and treatment, supervisory infrastructure as well as having robust policies and procedures that reflect current practice and knowledge. In the area of borderline personality disorder the compilation of policies and procedures goes a long way to enabling good practice to occur.

Medicolegal inquiry into whether there has been a breech of duty of care will include the following questions. Was there a forseeable risk? What is a reasonable response? What is a reasonable standard of practice? Frequently with this client group there is a forseeable risk and the question then turns to whether the magnitude of the forseeable risk was reasonably assessed and whether the clinical response was appropriate to the level of forseeable risk. The appropriateness of the clinical response will include the type and intensity of intervention. Effective treatment sometimes involves counter-intuitive actions such as discharging from hospital a client who is still expressing suicidal ideation. The assessment and treatment needs to be carefully thought through and documented. Medicolegal inquiry will want to see that there was a principled process of decision-making and that a clear rationale is documented for taking a particular pathway. In working with the chronic suicidality of people meeting diagnostic criteria for borderline personality disorder, there is no risk-free pathway.

What is required is a documented risk–benefit analysis as to why a particular pathway was considered to be, on balance, the best way of minimizing the risk and in the client's overall best interest. This may include choosing a pathway which entails higher short-term risk (such as discharge from hospital) in order to minimize long-term or overall risk. Other factors include balancing the ethical framework of the duty to do good with the duty to do no harm. Iatrogenic effects of treating people who meet diagnostic criteria for borderline personality disorder are well recognized. Maximizing safety needs to be balanced with treating the client in an environment and manner that will encourage client learning. For example, custodial interventions such as use of one to one observation and the use of the mental health act, and to a lesser degree hospitalization, increase immediate safety but decrease opportunities for the client to learn how to manage their risk and keep themselves safe. Protecting the client from suicidal actions needs to be balanced with assisting the client to learn alternative ways of dealing with distress other than suicide. These are all factors in the planning and assessment for crises with each client. Staff who are clear about their clinical responsibilities, are supported by the organization and have the tools to deliver the service to the client are more likely to enter into the relationship or interaction with the client in a therapeutic manner.

Clinicians from time to time have the difficult task of appearing before a coronial, professional or other system of inquiry. Any medicolegal inquiry will explore whether the necessary factual information was gathered, what decisions were made and what those decisions were based on. They will want evidence in the client file to back up the statements.

Most complaints arise out of allegations of poor professional judgement leading to claims of negligence. Demonstrating that practice was of a reasonable standard of care refutes negligence. Obtaining a second opinion, peer review specific to the client and presenting the clinical material to forums set up for complex clinical situations will be objective measures of the clinician checking out the reasonable practitioner standard. A reasonable standard of care will assume keeping abreast of current clinical developments. Different jurisdictions have distinct legal terminology and frameworks influencing clinician practice, which clinicians need to be aware of.

An understanding of the medicolegal interface, including terminology, contributes to proactively preparing the clinician for the possibility of a complaint. Having knowledge is empowering and contributes to clinicians taking necessary professionally indicated risks to enhance client outcome, despite the inevitable anxiety involved. Other measures that are helpful are: ensuring a risk–benefit analysis is done, widening and sharing the risk with the client, family and friends, clinical director, organizational lawyer and peer review group. Some of these actions are obviously harder to ensure in crisis situations but even here a second opinion can almost always be attained with a five-minute telephone call. Litigation is thought to be correlated with clients being surprised by the unexpected (Gutheil 1998). Informing and orientating the client (and, if applicable, relatives/friends) to treatment decreases this risk.

Thorough documentation is critical. Documentation will include a risk–benefit analysis and the reasons a particular pathway was considered to be in the client's best interest. Known risks, advantages and disadvantages of different pathways will have been thoroughly noted and the reasons why a particular pathway was chosen (e.g. risks and benefits of discharge or staying in hospital longer). Acute or chronic suicidality and short-term versus long-term risks and gains, if relevant to the decision-making will be noted. Documentation will include clinical judgement in action. For example "While there is a calculated risk in this hospital discharge, the treatment team, and Dr. A who provided an external second opinion, believe the risks of staying in hospital (regression, reinforcing self-concepts of helplessness and incompetence) outweigh the risks of discharge. Benefits include supporting autonomy and consequent self-esteem, and reinforcing concepts of self-capacity and competence. The risks have been discussed with the client who appears competent to understand the issues and also the client's relatives etc." Involvement of the client, relatives/friends, peers, supervisor, second opinion/s, and expert opinion will be noted. This will demonstrate that the clinician was mindful of not acting alone in what may be an inherently risk-filled situation.

Fictitious clinical vignette

Your client periodically continues to get very angry with her partner. She expresses a fear that she might take an axe to him if another situation arises with him. The partner is not at immediate risk. She advises you, that due to your unwillingness to prescribe Valium or have Valium prescribed for her, you will be responsible if she kills him.

Fictitious clinical vignette

A client advises you that one of the inpatient night staff slapped her face. She says this happened after she got up at 3 am. and put music on in the lounge. An argument followed as to whether this was going to disturb other patients. She says she got angry, and announced she was leaving the ward and went to the door which was locked (standard procedure at night for security reasons). The staff member arrived and there was a physical engagement around opening and not opening the door and this included him slapping her on the face, she says. She says she doesn't want him punished because he is a nice person who just lost his cool. She asks you whether you believe her and what you are going to do with the information.

Professionally indicated risk-taking

Staff anxiety in any mental health organization is directly proportional to how recently the **** hit the fan (ie a poor client outcome led to an inquiry or was reported in the media)
(Workshop participant commenting on professional anxiety in treating
 people meeting diagnostic criteria for borderline personality disorder)

I know what the right clinical decision is, but I am going to look after myself.
(Workshop participant commenting about
defensive practice at the expense of client outcome)

I think sometimes when doctors and nurses try and protect themselves
they're not really making decisions in the best interest of the patient.
(clinician quoted in: O'Brien and Flote 1997)

Historically in mental health there was a paucity of evidence-based effective treatment, mental health professionals practised in an environment which had few quality assurance systems in place and individual practitioners had little visibility. These factors led to varied methods and standards of practice, and on occasions, abuse of clients. This has appropriately changed with increasing visibility, accountability, peer review and other quality assurance programs. There has been an increase in consumer complaints and heightened media visibility. Clinicians have responded with increased concern about the quality of their work. This constructive concern is now sometimes being replaced, in the treatment of people meeting diagnostic criteria for borderline personality disorder, by a "culture of fear" leading to defensive practices that are destructive in many ways, particularly to client outcome. Recent risk assessment guidelines have recognized the issue:

> In order to achieve therapeutic gain, it is sometimes necessary to take risks. A strategy of total risk avoidance, could lead to excessively restricted management, which may in itself be damaging to the individual.
>
> (Ministry of Health 1998)

It is well recognized that provision of effective treatment for people meeting diagnostic criteria for borderline personality disorder requires decision-making which entails risk, including that of suicide. One of the core features of successful outcomes is that clients increasingly take on responsibility for themselves, including their treatment. Clients deteriorate or regress when clinicians take on excessive responsibility. Determining the amount of responsibility clinicians should take requires considerable skill, is individualized for each client and varies over time, often rapidly. There is an absence of clearly defined guidelines as to how active a clinician should be and how much responsibility a clinician should take, in response to a client's suicidal statements. Organizations and individuals may hold an illusion that there are clear guidelines and thereby set up unattainable expectations for clinicians to achieve.

People meeting diagnostic criteria for borderline personality disorder have a high rate of suicide and make suicidal statements when they are seriously considering killing themselves. Alongside this, suicidal statements are also used as a form of communication (Dawson 1988; Dawson and MacMillan 1993). Graham (personal communication 1998), an ex-consumer who set up a successful consumer-driven treatment program, says she used to tell her therapist she was about to kill herself so that she could have more time with her therapist. Once a pattern has emerged that suicidal statements are being used as communication, then it is likely that part of a successful treatment package will require the clinician responding to such suicidal statements in a manner encouraging the client to more constructive ways of communicating. This does not mean not responding to suicidal statements at all, but a judicious response to the client's distress at the time. This may take the form of collaboratively exploring what the client may do about their distress. Clinician responsiveness to more adaptive communications of distress from the client at other times will communicate to the client that they do not have to be suicidal to be responded to. Distinguishing between life-threatening and non life-threatening suicidal statements is a difficult and inexact task which Stone (1993) states is enhanced by clinical experience, supervision and knowledge of the literature on suicide risk.

Acute versus chronic suicide risk and short-term versus long-term risk/gain (see rest of section "The legal environment" in Part 4 and section "Assessment" in Part 2) are concepts likely to be discussed in medicolegal deliberations. Clinicians treating people meeting diagnostic criteria for borderline personality disorder, generally, need to be more interventionistic in the acute suicide as opposed to the chronic suicide situation. In the chronic suicide situation, a comprehensive treatment needs to be offered, alongside the recognition that being as interventionistic as in the acute suicide situation, may in fact, make the situation worse. To statistically increase the likelihood of the client being alive in the long term, one might need to make decisions that could increase the possibility of suicide in the short term.

The use of the term professionally indicated short-term risk-taking refers to a solid thorough decision-making process where risk assessment considers the balance of short-term and long-term risk and leans in the direction of increasing short-term risk in order to minimize overall risk. Professionally indicated short-term risk-taking involves the assessment of the nature and level of clinician and organization responses to self-harm and suicidality, that will be in the client's best interest. This is a clinical judgement based on knowledge of the client. Professionally indicated short-term risk-taking is a concept that can be applied in varying degrees to decision-making. Decisions will include which clients it might apply to, at what juncture in treatment it may apply, the level of clinician activity, the nature of clinician activity (balancing support and self-responsibility) and the level of short and long-term risk to take.

A professionally indicated short-term risk-taking approach synthesizes cross-sectional and longitudinal views. Crises need to be survived and also are valuable opportunities for learning about and changing chronic patterns, including alternatives to suicide and self-harm as ways of dealing with distress. Crises are opportunities for the client to work, with clinician support, on how to reduce their own risk and keep themselves safe. The client is supported and encouraged in their efforts to monitor and manage their own distress and safety. The client will be warmly engaged with and assisted to learn new positive coping strategies and be invited to maximize competence. The clinician's goal is to help, assist and aid client autonomy, self-responsibility and self-capacity. The goal is to decrease suicidal behaviour and to decrease the likelihood of intentional or accidental death.

There are ways of building structures into local systems that encourage clinicians to take professionally indicated risks. These structures can concurrently improve client outcome, protect clinicians from medicolegal risk and widen and share risks involved. Such structures include discussion with the client, client's significant support people, colleagues including peer review groups, clinical directors and organizational lawyers. Robinson (personal communication 1998) gives the example of an acute inpatient unit, where a standard cautious approach prevailed. An alternative clinical approach, which entailed some risk was developed, in line with developing clinical thinking. This risk was managed by every initial clinical plan being reviewed and supported by the clinical director, organization lawyer and a psychiatrist peer review group before being put in place. Clinicians may argue that there is insufficient time for such an intensive process. Whilst this requires intensive proactive input, it will probably be less time-consuming in the long run and also improve outcome.

Organizations that support clinicians who have practised according to reasonable professional standards, when taking professionally indicated risks, improve overall client outcome. When clinicians believe they can/ought, or their organization expects them to prevent somebody who is chronically suicidal from killing himself or herself, they may well practise in an iatrogenic manner. Typical examples may include prolonged hospitalization, lengthy one to one observation of the client and frequent or lengthy use of mental health legislation. This is a well-recognized phenomenon, but the environment clinicians work in often encourages the continuation of these practices. Relevant organizations include mental health providers, consumer organizations, mental health professional bodies and colleges, legal professionals, coroners, police, government health departments and the media.

Expectations of people and organizations need to be consistent across various conditions that have similar mortality rates. Stone's study (1989, 1990a, 1990b, 1993) suggested that those people meeting diagnostic criteria for the most severe forms of borderline personality disorder (and not treated with the evidence-based treatments now available) might have a five-year survival rate in the vicinity of 50%. This is comparable to people with Stage 3A breast cancer (fixed metastases to lymph nodes) (Lippman 1998) and malignant melanoma metastatic to regional nodes (Sober, Koh, Tran and Washington 1998). Fifty percent of people with acute renal failure die (Brady and Brenner 1998) and 10% of people with congestive heart failure with "mild left ventricular dysfunction and symptoms" will die per year (Braunwald 1998). Clinicians working in these fields are not regularly vilified for failure to save lives – the mortality rate is seen as a function of the disorder being treated.

Professionally indicated risk-taking can be enhanced by local clinicians, local organizations, organizational structures and key people external to the organization as listed in the following table.

Systems enabling professionally indicated risk-taking

Individual clinician

- Client
- Family and friends
- Second opinion (several if necessary)
- Documentation
- Reasonable practitioner standard

Local organization

- Supports professionally indicated risk-taking
  - Consumer groups
  - Clinical director
  - Manager
  - Lawyer
  - Other stakeholders (emergency, medical and surgical departments)

Organizational structure to process risk

- Policies and guidelines
- Peer review group
- Complex clinical situations forum (credibility to hold/support risk-filled decisions)

External to the Organization

- Professional organizations (colleges etc.)
- Central Government
  - Funders
  - Health departments
- Legal Profession
  - Coroners
  - Lawyers
- Police
- Media

The following pages are a collection of quotes from both consumers and clinicians around the issues of acute versus chronic suicide risk, short-term versus long-term risk, responsibility and communication behaviour.

Professionally indicated risk-taking
Acute vs chronic suicide risk/gain

Gutheil (1985)

The central issue in acute suicidal state is a matter of despair, guilt and a consequent, usually short lived emergency state that requires immediate intervention. In contrast, the chronic suicidal state represents a seriously disturbed yet consistent mode of relating to objects in the environment. In this condition the central issue is the assumption of responsibility by the patient for his or her own life and its fate. The requisite interventions are not, as in an acute state, directed towards shepherding patients through a short term crisis until the self destructive press has passed, by somatic or psychotherapeutic approaches.

Milton and Banfai (1999)

The traditional therapeutic manoeuvres used to manage acute suicidality may actually reinforce destructive interpersonal dynamics in the case of chronic suicidality, causing a malignant regression whereby hospitalization worsens the suicidal risk. The clinician who engages in paternalistic and directive interventions may provoke understandable oppositional behaviour, testing of limits, dependency and further suicidal behaviour.

Paris (1993)

To be derailed by chronic suicidality is to lose sight of the real work of psychotherapy. Paradoxically only by tolerating its chronicity can borderline suicidality be successfully treated.

Maltsberger (1994)

The truth of the matter is that taking calculated risks with patients who suffer from chronic suicidal pathology is perfectly

Professionally indicated risk-taking
Acute vs chronic suicide risk/gain *(cont.)*

defensible from a legal point of view. Though it is true that suicide, even under the best clinical circumstances, may arouse the lawyers, releasing a suicidal patient from the hospital, or declining to admit a patient to the hospital, need not constitute negligence if the decisions are made in the correct way and if they are correctly documented"

Cantor and McDermott (1994)

The following measures are suggested when dealing with the chronically suicidal from the perspective of self (legal) defence. First, the chronic risk and its management should be discussed with the patient and this discussion documented; Second, it should be documented that the chronic nature of the suicidal state warrants a certain approach; Third, it may be desirable to inform and involve the family; a further option is to get a second opinion.

Fine and Sansone (1990)

Approaches to managing "acute" suicidal situations may be inappropriate for the "chronic" suicidal states of many borderlines.

Professionally indicated risk-taking
Short-term vs long-term risk/gain

Linehan (1993a)

... in working with chronically suicidal individuals, there will be times when reasonably high short-term risks must be taken to produce long-term benefits.

Gutheil (1985)

To put this in crude as possible terms, the evaluators choice, largely by hindsight, appears to lie between two outcomes – a concrete dead body and the rather abstract notion of personal growth. No wonder the decision is so charged with anxiety.

Professionally indicated risk-taking
Short-term vs long-term risk/gain (cont.)

The crisis recovery service (undated)

The Maudsley, The Bethlehem and Maudsley NHS trust

It follows from an approach which insists on individuals taking responsibility for their own behaviour that risks to the short-term safety of residents may need to be taken in the interests of their long-term safety and health.

Williams (1998)

The most important thing is, do not hospitalize a person with borderline personality disorder for any more than 48 hours. My self-destructive episodes – one leading right into another – came only after my first and subsequent hospital admissions, after I learned the system was usually obligated to respond. . . . I would never have the life I have today if I had continued to get the intermittent reinforcement of hospitalization.

Maltsberger (1994)

When we see that continued monitoring, vigilance, and preemptive anti-suicidal intervention is leading to the development of coercive bondage and psychotherapeutic stalemate, giving responsibility back to the patient for the decision whether to live or commit suicide becomes not only ethically defensible but ethically necessary. At such junctures, a restrictive course heightens the long term risk of suicide. Giving responsibility back to the patient, even though the immediate risk may increase for a time, can be the best hope.

Ministry of Health (1998)

In order to achieve therapeutic gain, it is sometimes necessary to take risks. A strategy of total risk avoidance, could lead to excessively restricted management, which may in itself be damaging to the individual.

Professionally indicated risk-taking
Short-term vs long-term risk/gain (cont.)

Linehan (1993a)

The therapist should remind the patient that calling after engaging in self-injurious behavior is not appropriate, and should instruct her to contact other resources (family, friends, emergency services). Except in very unusual circumstances, the conversation should then be terminated.

Jackson (1999)

I had learnt to access services by being at risk and you reinforce this if you over-respond. Focusing excessively on suicidality stopped me from focusing on the important things behind it and therefore prevented change.

Professionally indicated risk-taking
Responsibility

Dawson (1988; Dawson and MacMillan 1993)

I do not know what I have to offer ... but if you would like to come and talk with me ....

No-therapy therapy.

Everett and Nelson (1992)

I had read books and I had heard 50 million therapists say that I was the only one who could make myself happy. I finally understood. If I didn't like what was going on, I could change it. No one else was going to do it. Being responsible for myself is power.

Jackson (1999)

I really wanted someone to cure me and was irritated, to say the least, when it was suggested that I might, at least in part, be that someone. It took a long while and considerable conflict with

Professionally indicated risk-taking
Responsibility *(cont.)*

mental health services to realize that the answer lay within myself. With the wonderful benefit of hindsight, I now see that eventually coming to this realization was a major turning point in my treatment.

Graham (personal communication 1998)

As an ex-consumer who now works with consumers, I believe that each person should be held responsible for their own behaviours. The professional should work with utmost honesty and do whatever they can to help, but they should not be responsible for the client's behaviours. When a professional takes responsibility for their client's behaviour, they then develop a power struggle which they will not win.

Kroll (1993)

The foundation of therapy is that the therapist agrees to work with patients to help them make changes in their lives, not to be the provider of their emotional needs or to act as rescuer or the guarantor of their safety. The therapist simply cannot play these roles, and to try to do so is to court therapeutic disaster.

Professionally indicated risk-taking
Communication behaviour

Everett and Nelson (1992)

Anne: The only way I had gotten attention for years was to talk about doing something to myself and I thought well, it would work well here too. In fact, I thought it would be the only thing that would work. The reaction I got was that Barbara would not deal with me on that level...

Barbara: When feeling powerless and out of control, she used the only weapon she knew "I'm going to kill myself". Over the

Professionally indicated risk-taking Communication behaviour (cont.)

next few meetings, Anne and I explored her feelings regarding the suicide threats and the incidents of self-harm. ... We discussed how the formal mental health system (the hospital) was most vulnerable to her threats and that she was always bound to get a big reaction in that environment when she threatened suicide. We also looked at the downside of that reaction; the humiliation of restraints, the sense that the inpatient team really had no caring for her at all unless whipped into action by a threat or attempt and her sense that none of these reactions assuaged her aching feelings of loneliness or her frantic need for affection.

...

Anne: I remember that when my outpatient therapist was about to leave for her new job, I told her that I was really going to kill myself this time. She had me certified and dragged off to hospital. I told her I would never forgive her. It caused a rift between us that might never have been resolved. I did this to the only caring relationship in my life. ... I decided I would never again jeopardize a relationship by threatening suicide.

(Printed with the permission of the Center for Psychiatric Rehabilitation)

Graham (personal communication 1998)

I used to tell my therapist I was going to kill myself so that I could spend more time with her.

Jackson (personal communication 1999)

If I know that this worker here is going to respond to "I'm having a difficult day – could you support me" – I am going to use that line with them again. The problem comes when two hours later you go off duty and I know the only way I am going to get support from you is to say that "I have been suicidal all day and I am going to kill myself.

Note!

A willingness to take risk and to not take on too much responsibility for the client is not an invitation to avoid treatment or engage in practices that are laissez faire and without monitoring and quality assurance. A danger exists for clinicians to not see themselves as accountable, if the views expressed in this section are taken on superficially and poorly integrated. Decision-making involving risk is a carefully thought out process within a framework of current research and emerging clinical thinking.

Fictitious clinical vignette

Your client has made suicidal statements on fifteen occasions which have not resulted in an attempt to kill herself but have resulted in three overdoses, cutting her wrists superficially five times, deeply once, resulting in nerve damage, and once cutting her throat superficially. The clinical response to date has been to increase the therapeutic endeavours with increased clinician time and on four occasions, hospitalization. You feel you are in an un-therapeutic stalemate. Whilst she has not tried to kill herself in the past you believe this to be a distinct possibility at some point.

Two months earlier, you discussed with her, her family, your manager and your clinical director the possibility of changing the therapeutic strategy so as to not reinforce suicidal statements and self-harm. This would mean not increasing therapeutic input (including hospitalization) at times of suicidal statements or self-harm. Her parents complained to their MP who made inquiries of you, your clinical director and your manager. It was decided to make no fundamental changes to the therapeutic strategy.

You are anxious that if you don't fundamentally change the strategy this will lead to clinical deterioration, an increased chance in the long term of suicide, exhausting the resources of those trying to treat her, killing herself by accident and a deterioration in others' appraisal of you and the consequences to your self-esteem and career. You are anxious that if you do change the strategy that this will lead to her refusal to be involved with you, suicide as a direct result of the change, professional complaint to the MP, the media, your employer or professional body, a deterioration in others' appraisal of you and the consequences to your self-esteem and career.

Fictitious clinical vignette

You work on an acute inpatient ward where your client has been for 170 days. She has been on constant observation for 94 days. As soon as constant observations are stopped, she makes suicidal statements or self-harms. Most of the self-harm episodes are associated with suicidal statements inconsistent with the lack of lethality used. However, two self-harm episodes were difficult to interpret in terms of intended lethality. On one further occasion, her desire to die was ambivalent and her behaviour made sure that it was left to fate whether she lived or died. You believe that treatment is going nowhere. You are aware of reinforcing destructive behaviours but feel locked in by the knowledge that she is at risk of suicide. You believe she will have a high suicide risk whether you adopt a new, less restrictive approach or stay with the status quo. You are concerned about medicolegal consequences if you move to a less restrictive approach.

Clinical appropriateness of the use of mental health legislation

Expert opinion is in agreement that use of mental health legislation should be considered an unusual part of treatment. Mental health legislation is generally invoked when a client states acute intention to suicide. When the client makes contact with mental health services, indicates imminent suicide intention and then declines treatment measures to enhance safety, the clinician has to either take a risk of the client suiciding or force treatment by means of mental health legislation. Training, experience and knowledge of the literature assist the discrimination of life-threatening and non life-threatening suicidal statements (Stone 1993). Knowledge of the client will greatly assist in discriminating between these two states. If the client is not well known, it is wise to err on the side of caution. Like any other unusual treatment, use of mental health legislation needs to be monitored and locally peer reviewed.

The disadvantage of mental health legislation is that it runs completely counter to core principles upon which successful treatment is based. A core principle is that clients be responsible for their behaviour. The use of mental health legislation implies clinicians will assume responsibility for clients' behaviour. Use of mental health legislation increases the inevitable power struggle, is disempowering, decreases autonomy and self-sufficiency and increases passivity – the very opposite of treatment goals.

When the client is new to the system, the service might need to err on the conservative side until the picture becomes clearer. However, unless clinicians are vigilant, this can lead to a situation of repeated or ongoing use of mental health legislation because a precedent has been set which in the short term provokes the least staff anxiety.

If mental health legislation is used, wherever possible, it should be used, for as brief a period as possible – up to 72 hours. Clinicians should feel comfortable and supported to remove a person from mental health legislation within as little as a day if the imminent acute suicide risk has lessened.

Discharging a client from hospital frequently involves some continuing risk. A professional risk-benefit analysis will determine whether staying in hospital is a greater or lesser risk. Again, training needs to clarify the assessment of acute and chronic suicide risk and of short-term and long-term risk.

When people have more control of their treatment (especially the capacity to admit themselves for brief periods) and they are being "reached to" with resourcing (rather than being kept away at arm's length), then the whole issue of mental health legislation often melts away.

In summary

- There is significant medicolegal risk because of the possibility of suicide and complaints
- Clinicians need to practise according to a "reasonable practitioner standard"
- Demonstration of professional judgement based on a sound risk–benefit analysis in keeping with a "reasonable practitioner standard" will be used to refute a charge of negligence
- Obtaining a second (or more) opinion will indicate that there was checking of the "reasonable practitioner standard"
- The riskier the circumstance and the more radical the treatment approach, the more widely the clinician needs to seek out other opinion
- Different jurisdictions have distinct legal terminology and frameworks influencing clinician practice
- Thorough documentation is critical
- A "culture of fear" can exist with clinicians aware they are doing their clients a disservice by practising defensively

- If the client is and has been chronically suicidal (without an acute exacerbation), the clinician generally needs to be less interventionistic than with an acutely suicidal client
- To increase the likelihood of a client being alive in the long-term, one might need to make decisions whereby there is an increased possibility of suicide in the short-term
- There are ways of building structures into local systems encouraging clinicians to take professionally indicated risks. Such structures include discussion with the client, client's significant support people, colleagues, clinical directors and organizational lawyers
- Peer review will provide significant medicolegal protection thereby encouraging professionally indicated risk-taking
- There is international literature supporting the concepts of acute versus chronic suicide risk, short versus long-term risk-taking, responsibility and communication behaviour as important considerations in determining clinical decision-making around risk
- Decision-making involving risk is a carefully thought out process within a framework of current research and emerging clinical thinking
- Mental health legislation use is counter to the principle that the client is responsible for their behaviour and is likely to increase power struggles and decrease autonomy and self-sufficiency
- Mental health legislation needs to be considered an unusual part of treatment and subject to routine local peer review.

Part 5

Maintaining enthusiasm

Limit-setting

Literature over the last decade has legitimized the importance and appropriateness of limit-setting to prevent clinician burn-out (Adler 1993; Linehan 1993a; Young 1996a; Young 1996b). Limit-setting is appropriately used to increase clients' adaptive behaviours and interpersonal skills and has been written about extensively, however there has been little written on the legitimacy of limit-setting for the needs of the clinician. The culture of the health professions as "giving" and "caring" has discouraged the legitimate rights of clinicians to look after themselves. It is in the client's interest that clinicians look after themselves and set limits accordingly, as a burnt-out clinician who resents their client will not be therapeutic. Naming limit-setting as necessary for the clinician is associated with a more benevolent attitude towards the client. Therapists holding a "non-pejorative conceptualization" of people meeting diagnostic criteria for borderline personality disorder has been shown by Shearin and Linehan (1992) to be associated with better client outcomes measured by a decrease in client self-harm and suicide thoughts.

Limit-setting needs to be used sparingly, as it is a unilateral non-collaborative action. Limit-setting needs to be, wherever possible, in the context of a responsive, supportive and validating relationship. The clinician asks the client what they want and the clinician/system states what can or can't be delivered (Dawson 1988; Dawson and MacMillan 1993). Client and clinician then negotiate and discuss consequences if the clinician/system boundaries are breached.

When preparing to set a limit, clinicians need to be prepared for an escalation of behaviour as the client checks whether what is stated will be carried through. If clinicians are uncertain about their or the system's capacity to maintain the limit in the face of an escalation of behaviour, then it is best not to set the limit.

Intermittent reinforcement of the behaviour will otherwise occur, which is very difficult to alter.

Inappropriate limit-setting can sometimes be a result of the clinician being unable to constructively process their feelings for the client. For this reason, wherever possible, the clinician should delay limit-setting when angry with the client. It is important for clinicians to monitor their own limits, communicate these clearly to each client and to be aware of warning signs that their own limits are being reached. The greater care clinicians take of themselves, such as tending to physical, emotional and spiritual well-being, the broader and more flexible their limits are likely to be. Attention to caseload, supervision and consultation needs will have a similar effect.

Fictitious clinical vignette

You are looking forward to a long-awaited weekend holiday away. You know you need and deserve the break because of the difficult and heavy workload you have been carrying over the last couple of months. You finish work at 5 pm. Your friends/family are due to pick you up at 5.30 pm. directly from work, so you all can get away on your holiday as soon as possible. You have been seeing your client for 15 months, once/week initially and now once/fortnight, with frequent additional phone calls and the occasional extra session at times of crisis. Your client rings at 4.15 pm. As you are not available she leaves a message with the receptionist which your client says is essential you get before you go for the day. "Please ring A... urgently, she needs to speak to you – she says she is feeling suicidal – she sounded really distressed and agitated". You get the message at 4.45 pm. This is about the twentieth call like this. The crisis usually settles when you phone her back, occasionally you have scheduled an extra session and on two occasions you have arranged her admission because of the significant acute risk of suicide. You know she dislikes the people available for emergencies from 5 pm.

Fictitious clinical vignette

Your client has a history of deterioration at times when significant people in her life are not present. This deterioration manifests in many ways including self-harm and hospitalization. Six weeks ago her relationship with her partner broke up. Out of compassion and as a therapeutic endeavour to prevent deterioration, you have been seeing her twice/week instead of the previous once/week. You hoped the increased frequency would be temporary but there is no indication that this will be the case in the near future. In addition she telephones about twice a week acutely distressed. You telephone her back at a time of relative convenience for you and after about half an hour she is sufficiently settled. This involves an extra two hours work/week of a very difficult nature, on top of your extremely heavy workload. The emergency team ring you at home on the weekend to get advice. You believe there is a chronic risk of suicide, which is intensified currently. You believe she is likely to see any reduction of input from yourself as rejecting and punitive. You are exhausted physically (not sleeping well because of worry) and emotionally. You are beginning to doubt whether you were cut out for this work and you know you are burning out. Hospitalization of the client in the past has created as many if not more problems than it has helped with.

Preventing clinician burn-out

Work in this area is challenging. There is potential for clinician resentment, bitterness and exhaustion alongside the potential for meaningful, satisfying and rich experiences. The clinician may "explode", "shrivel up" or quietly burn out if overwhelmed with demands exceeding resources and personal capacity. Alternatively, the clinician may be enhanced, enriched and energized if sufficiently on top of the situation.

Successful outcomes are likely to be the major factor in maintaining enthusiasm. We may need to remind ourselves and our colleagues of those successes, particularly at times of difficulty. Holding a long-term perspective and being mindful of small gains is also likely to be beneficial. The more knowledge we have of setting up treatment which will enhance successful outcomes, the more the balance is shifted away from burn-out towards satisfaction.

Another major factor in maintaining enthusiasm is the value and status given to the work by ourselves and our colleagues. In the past some clinicians were told they were engaging in this work to meet their own needs or that the client group were not deserving of resources ("bring it on themselves"; "worried well"). Compare that with "These clients really deserve the best we have to offer. You are working in an important and extremely difficult area, which requires immense personal and professional skills, and with considerable professional risk. I am glad that there are people like you who want to do this work. I would like to support you in your job, so let me know how I can assist you". Over the last twenty years work in the area of schizophrenia has changed from relatively low to relatively high status. Working in the area of borderline personality disorder requires the same status.

Being mindful of one's own emotional needs is another critical determinant. The goal is for clinicians to have and maintain the enthusiasm so frequently seen with new graduates. This requires an awareness of emotional pitfalls, support from experienced, skilled colleagues and a perspective of maintaining ourselves over a lengthy career. What is good for the clinician is usually good for current and future clients. Clients will not benefit from an apathetic, de-energized clinician, especially if the client is aware that they are contributing to overwhelming that person. Factors that will decrease the likelihood of burn-out are listed in the table below.

Preventing clinician burn-out

Effective treatment structures

- Team structure
- Team culture
- Individualized clinical plans
- Conceptual frameworks to guide treatment

Workload

- Reasonable workload
- Some clinicians prefer to limit the number of people meeting diagnostic criteria for borderline personality disorder that they provide treatment for
- Some clinicians prefer to have an exclusive workload and focus on people meeting diagnostic criteria for borderline personality disorder, provided workload is not excessive

Realistic expectations

- Clinicians expect to feel powerless, at times
- Clinicians/organizations acknowledge the possibility of suicide despite competent practice

Preventing clinician burn-out *(cont.)*

- Clinicians and organizations be practically and emotionally prepared for a complaint

Personal

- Self-validation of the importance of the work
- Finding personal meaning in the work
- Mindful of personal limits
- Tending to physical, emotional, and spiritual needs outside the work context

Regular ongoing supervision

- Supervision which is focused, skilled and meets the clinician's needs (see "Supervision" section)

Professional development

- Training (initial and ongoing) commensurate with the difficulty of the work
- Supervision as ongoing training
- Networking
- Stimulation by keeping abreast of recent developments (literature, conferences)
- Evaluation which demonstrates efficacy of one's work is energizing and validating

Culture of support

- Limit-setting to prevent burn-out and to maintain positivity for the client is legitimate
- Availability of skilled senior staff to provide second opinion at short notice
- Sharing responsibility with family, team, institution, manager, colleagues, lawyer
- Culture which validates the work
- Institutional/system support for professionally indicated risk-taking

Preventing clinician burn-out *(cont.)*

- ◆ Satisfactory indemnity insurance (for legal support should a complaint arise requiring legal assistance)
- ◆ Supportive peer review systems in place

The considerable flexible personal attributes required of the clinician need to be valued and affirmed. The clinician needs to have a wide range of personal qualities that they can draw upon, in the client's interest, as the need arises. The table opposite lists some of these qualities. Not only are numerous qualities required, many of these qualities are on opposite sides of a continuum as listed in the table. For example, toughness and firmness as well as nurturing and compassion are required. This requires considerable flexibility of the clinician for the client's moment-to-moment needs.

Other clinician attributes include relative comfort with verbal anger, sensitivity to separation experiences and a generally positive world-view. A high tolerance for emotional pain will enable the clinician to recognize, validate and empathize with the pain and not deny, numb or get overwhelmed by the pain (Pilkonis 1997). A willingness to hold a position in the face of challenge requires a certain courage and fortitude and needs to be balanced with a capacity to invite and respond to feedback. Allen (1997) explored similarities between four different treatment models and summarizes:

> Therapists present themselves as ... unafraid of the patient's anger, neediness or anxiety; and as unwilling to attack the patient in the face of provocation. They do not rush in to "take care of" the patient in an infantilizing manner. They are in tune with and respectful of their own needs. Furthermore, they are relentlessly respectful of the patient's suffering, abilities, and values. They communicate an expectation that the patient will be able to behave reasonably and cooperatively, and they play to the patient's strengths. They presume that a patient with BPD has the ability to go through the therapy process like any other patient.

Clinician attributes that might be non-therapeutic include a poor capacity to act decisively, limited capacity for self-reflection,

Clinician attributes

Nurturing/Compassionate	Tough/Firm
Nurturing/Compassionate	Limit-setting capacity
Nurturing/Compassionate	Capacity to tolerate not being liked
Sensitive	Firm
See, hear and know pain	Know how to step away from pain
Flexible	Centred (Linehan 1993a)
Flexible	Firm
Flexible boundary	Firm boundary
Generous to others	Generous to self/Self-nurturing
Going the extra mile for others	Self-nurturing
Accepting client and self	Expecting change in client and self (Linehan, 1993a)
Ability to know one's powerlessness	Ability to know one's power
Comfortable with own powerlessness	Comfortable with own power
Capacity to know own weaknesses	Courage to trust own strengths
Tolerate ambiguity	Ordered, disciplined
Tolerate paradox	Ordered, disciplined
Emotional skills	Cognitive skills
Self-reflection skills	Skills to act
Patience – capacity to wait	Capacity to act
Function as a team person	Function autonomously

rigidity, excessive self-doubt and poor awareness of one's limitations. The inability to set limits and look after one's own needs and boundary issues can manifest in overly intimate, invasive or distancing behaviour.

Supervision

Supervision provides an essential "safe space for clinicians to think and reflect on, rather than deny and flee from, problems and feelings" (Owen 1998). Working with suicidal people who frequently want assistance that can't be provided and turn down offers of what can be provided, may lead to feelings of powerlessness, anger and despair. Supervision provides a space where these feelings can be recognized, normalized and worked with, to the benefit of client and clinician. "Supervision benefits the therapist by offering a relationship which aims to guide, mentor, inspire, emotionally support and develop insight and understanding in the therapist" (NZAP 1997).

Supervision may be more educational with inexperienced clinicians and more reflective for more experienced clinicians. Clinicians do not feel safe with overly critical supervisors and are bored with overly supportive supervisors who do not challenge and assist the clinician to be more skilful. Supervisees describe the best supervisors as those who flexibly support or challenge as needs arise. Supervision tends to work best when there is a good fit between supervisor and supervisee. For this reason it is beneficial for the supervisee to have a choice of supervisors. Line hierarchy supervision in an organization is often appropriate, but limits the emotional safety of the supervisory space as the supervisee is less likely to share vulnerabilities and weaknesses with someone who could influence their career. Horizontal or peer supervision provides greater safety but doesn't meet the needs of hierarchical supervision.

Supervision in the effective evidence-based research of Linehan *et al.* and Stevenson/Meares was an essential part of the treatment package. Supervision is essential to effective treatment outcomes and not a luxury to be added when possible. Clinicians who have a significant part of their work with people meeting diagnostic criteria for borderline personality disorder need to have regular weekly supervision.

Various possible tasks of supervision are listed in the table following.

Supervision

Assists the clinician to maintain the "middle road" in client interactions

Objectivity – emotionally less engaged perspective

Therapist blind spots

Different perspective – "third eye"

Assists a culture of remaining open to critique

Place to tend to feelings including anger and aversion to client

Place to decrease relating to only a part dimension of the client

Place for clinician to develop and maintain realistic expectations of themselves, community and client

Place to validate and give status to the work done

Place to prevent or minimize invalidation of therapist by colleagues

Place to prevent or minimize invalidation of clients

Support and encouragement for clinician

Supervision as one of the best forms of ongoing training

Focused, skilled supervision is an essential part of the treatment package (consistent with evidence-based treatment outcomes)

Words of hope from clients

A word of advice to mental health professionals that cannot be stressed too strongly: don't define people with borderline personality disorder too strongly by any textbook limitations you have read. I have exceeded my doctor's expectations for improvement and he doesn't know how far I can progress. For the most part I've stayed out of the hospital, maintain long-term full time employment, live independently, have a motor vehicle, and plan to pursue further educational opportunities. If I – as one of the most chronic, regular, persistent visitors to emergency rooms in my community between the late 1980s and early 1990s, and as one of the most chronic hospital escapees, and as someone who was written off and told so – could triumph over borderline personality disorder to this extent, I'm sure other people with the disorder can at least improve the quality of their lives.

(Williams 1998; Reprinted with permission of the American Psychiatric Association)

For all that I yelled and screamed and gave you a hard time, and bothered you at home, and for all my joshing you for your psychiatric bullshit, the fact is that you always stayed with me, you never deserted me or exploited me, and even though you enraged me most of the time, I have to admire your honesty and stick-to-itness. I used to think you were the most brilliant and wonderful therapist; I'm not so sure about that any more. But I do know that you were straight with me, you stuck by the rules we set, you were always professional, and mostly... mostly I am feeling so much better. My life is reasonably okay now.

(Rockland 1992; Reprinted with the permission of Guilford Press)

I started self-harming at the age of 11, came into contact with mental health services at 18 and had over 50 psychiatric admissions, many under mental health legislation and many for several months. My coping skills were severely lacking, and I was genuinely unable to tolerate the incredible pain I felt. I have held almost every diagnosis in the book and have tried most medications that exist, with little or no success. My situation was, in my mind, desperate and without hope. The first step in my recovery was being accurately diagnosed followed by a clinical plan. Relationships of trust with mental health clinicians slowly developed and I began to use available support. I now use mental health services to prevent a crisis rather than diffuse one. Instead of, "I am going to kill myself", it is now, "I am finding things a bit difficult, could you help me to find ways to help myself." I am now living a life again. After many years on a benefit I am working, dealing with a stressful family situation, and leading an active social life. I have not reached all my goals yet, but it is some time since I self-harmed or even seriously considered it. For the first time in my life I am genuinely living a life with long-term goals and a vision for the future, something I didn't have before and didn't think was possible.

(Jackson 1999)

The past fifteen months have been a time of great personal struggle for me. I have lost six family members and friends to death, and helped several others through serious illnesses. One beloved family member died in my arms. My scarred, but not bloody, arms. As I sat down to write this editorial, I realized that despite the incredible stresses of the past year, I have not cut, burned nor bruised myself. I have not even considered doing so. In the midst of profound grief, shock, outrage, and fear, I did not consider SIV (self-inflicted violence). I did not need to. I had not made a promise to anyone, including myself to avoid SIV. I have always believed that if I need to cut, I need to cut. Survival always comes first. But I also can attest to the possibility of living without SIV, even in immensely difficult times. One after another, unexpectedly for most, I lost many I loved. My own healing had evolved to a place, however, wherein I did not consider SIV to help me cope with very deep and raw emotions and extremely difficult decisions. Through my own experiences of a healing relationship, by learning empathy, respect for and trust in myself, I had arrived in this strong and powerful place. Without question, life without SIV is preferable to that with it. It was not controlling SIV that led me to the freedom I now have, but outgrowing the need for it. I am truly grateful for all the healing relationships I have had, including that with myself, which have brought me to this new place. To say that the journey has been worth the effort is truly an understatement.

(Mazelis 1997/1998; Reprinted with the permission of The Cutting Edge)

In summary

- Limit-setting for the clinician's needs is legitimate to enable the clinician not to burn-out and retain positivity for the client
- Successful outcomes are likely to be the biggest factor maintaining enthusiasm
- Holding a long-term perspective and being mindful of small gains provides a realistic framework on which to measure success
- Value and status given to the client, clinician and the work will help sustain enthusiasm
- What is good for the clinician is usually good for current and future clients
- Clients will not benefit from an apathetic, de-energized clinician
- Burn-out can be prevented by an effective team structure and culture, reasonable workload, realistic expectations,

appropriate training, ongoing supervision and the clinician tending to their emotional, physical and spiritual needs
- The considerable flexible personal attributes required of the clinician need to be valued and affirmed
- Supervision provides an essential "safe space for clinicians to think and reflect on ... problems and feelings" (Owen 1998)
- Supervision aims to inspire
- Good supervision flexibly supports or challenges as needs arise
- Supervision is an essential part of the treatment package, not a luxury to be added when possible
- Clients who have had successful outcomes create hope for clients and clinicians

Guided reading

Diagnosis

Gunderson, J. (2001) Differential diagnosis: overlaps, subtleties and treatment implications. Chapter 2 in *Borderline personality disorder: a clinical guide*. American Psychiatric Press, Washington DC, pp. 35–62.

Comorbidity

Zanarini, M.C., Frankenberg, F.R., Dubo, E.D. *et al.* (1998) Axis I comorbidity of borderline personality disorder. *American Journal of Psychiatry*, **155**, 1733–1739.

Zanarini, M.C., Frankenberg, F.R., Dubo, E.D., Sickel, A.E., Trikha, A., Levin, A. *et al.* (1998) Axis II comorbidity of borderline personality disorder. *Comprehensive Psychiatry*, **39**, 296–302.

Psychosis

Umgvari, G.S., Mullen, P.E. (2000) Reactive psychoses revisited. *Australian and New Zealand Journal of Psychiatry*, **34**, 458–467.

Rating scales

Millon, T., Davis, R. (2000) The assessment of personality. In *Personality disorders in modern life*. John Wiley, New York, pp. 82–86.

Epidemiology

Swartz, M., Blazer, D., George, L., Winfield, I. (1990) Estimating the prevalence of borderline personality disorder in the community. *Journal of Personality Disorders*, **4**, 257–272.

Health resource use

Gabbard, O.G., Lazar, S.G., Hornberger, J., Spiegel D. (1997) The economic impact of psychotherapy: a review. *American Journal of Psychiatry*, **154**, 147–155.

Prognosis

Paris, J. (1993) The treatment of borderline personality disorder in light of the research on its long term outcome. *Canadian Journal of Psychiatry*, **38**(S1), S28–S34.

Aetiology

Zanarini, M.C., Frankenburg, F.R. (1997) Pathways to the development of borderline personality disorder. *Journal of Personality Disorders*, **11**, 93–104.

Biology

Silk, K.R. ed. (1998) *Biology of personality disorders.* Review of Psychiatry, Vol 17. American Psychiatric Press, Washington DC.

Treatment outcome research – psychosocial

Bateman, A., Fonagy, P. (1999) Effectiveness of partial hospitalisation in the treatment of borderline personality disorder: a randomised controlled trial. *American Journal of Psychiatry*, **156**, 1563–1569.

Koons, C.R., Robins, C.J., Tweed, I.L., Lynch, T.R., Gonzalez, A.M., Morse, J.Q. *et al.* (2001) Efficacy of dialectical behaviour therapy in women veterans with borderline personality disorder. *Behavior Therapy*, **32**, 371–390.

Linehan, M.M., Armstrong, H., Suarez, L., Allmon, D. (1991) Cognitive-behavioural treatment of chronically parasuicidal borderline patients. *Archives of General Psychiatry*, **48**, 1060–1064.

Linehan, M.M., Schmidt, H., Dimeff, L.A., Kanter, J., Comtois, K.A. (1999) Dialectical behavior therapy for patients with borderline personality disorder and drug dependence. *American Journal on Addiction*, **8**, 279–292.

Meares, R., Stevenson, J., Comerford, A. (1999) Psychotherapy with borderline patients: a comparison between treated and untreated cohorts. *Australian and New Zealand Journal of Psychiatry*, **33**, 467–472.

Munroe-Blum, H., Marziali, E. (1995) A controlled trial of short term group treatment for borderline personality disorder. *Journal of Personality Disorders*, **9**, 190–198.

Stevenson, J., Meares, R. (1992) An outcome study of psychotherapy for patients with borderline personality disorder. *American Journal of Psychiatry*, **149**, 358–362.

Turner, R.M. (2000) Naturalistic evaluation of dialectical behavior therapy-oriented treatment for borderline personality disorder. *Cognitive and Behavioral Practice*, **7**, 413–419.

Treatment outcome research and opinion – pharmacological

Gabbard, G.O. (2000). Combining medication with psychotherapy in the treatment of personality disorders. Chapter 3 in: *Review of Psychiatry*, Vol. 19(3). Gunderson, J.G., Gabbbard, G.O. eds. American Psychiatric Press, Washington DC, pp. 65–94.

Solloff, P.H. (2000) Psychopharmacology of borderline personality disorder. *Psychiatric Clinics of North America*, **23**(1), 169–192.

Woo-Ming, A.M., Siever, L.J. (1998) Psychopharmacological treatment of personality disorders. Chapter 28 in: *A guide to treatments that work*. Nathan, P.E., Gorman, J.M. eds. Oxford University Press, New York, pp. 544–553.

Psychodynamic

Adler, G. (1993) The psychotherapy of core borderline psychopathology. *American Journal of Psychotherapy*, **47**, 194–205.

Main, T.F. (1957) The ailment. *British Journal of Medical Psychology*, **30**, 129–145.

Meares, R. (1994) Psychotherapeutic treatments of severe personality disorder. *Current Opinion in Psychiatry*, **7**, 245–248.

Cognitive therapy

Beck, A., Freeman, A. (1990) Borderline personality disorder. Chapter 9 in: *Cognitive therapy for personality disorders*. Guilford, New York.

DBT

Linehan, M. (1993) *Cognitive behavioral treatment of borderline personality disorder*. Guilford Press, New York.

Linehan, M. (1993) *Skills training manual for treating borderline personality disorder*. Guilford Press, New York.

Schema-focused therapy

Young, J.E. (1994) *Cognitive therapy for personality disorders: a schema focused approach*. Professional Resource Exchange, Sarasota.

Relationship management

Dawson, D., MacMillan, H. (1993) *Relationship management of the borderline patient: from understanding to treatment*. Brunner/Mazel, New York.

Dawson, D.F.L. (1993) Relationship management and the borderline patient. *Canadian Family Physician*, **39**, 833–839.

Cognitive analytic therapy

Ryle, A. (1997) The structure and development of borderline personality disorder: a proposed model. *British Journal of Psychiatry*, **170**, 82–87.

Motivational interviewing

Miller, W.R., Rollnick, S. (1991) *Motivational interviewing – preparing people to change addictive behavior.* Guilford Press, New York.

Rehabilitation

Links, P.S. (1993) Psychiatric rehabilitation model for borderline personality disorder. *Canadian Journal of Psychiatry,* **38**, S35–S38.

Nehls, N., Diamond, R.J. (1993) Developing a systems approach to caring for persons with borderline personality disorder. *Community Mental Health Journal,* **29**, 161–172.

Integration

Allen, D.M. (1997) Techniques for reducing therapy-interfering behavior in patients with borderline personality disorder: similarities in four diverse treatment paradigms. *Journal of Psychotherapy Practice and Research,* **6**, 25–35.

Bateman, A.W. (1997) Borderline personality disorder and psychotherapeutic psychiatry: an integrative approach. *British Journal of Psychotherapy,* **13**, 489–498.

Livesley, W.J. (2000) A practical treatment approach to the treatment of patients with borderline personality disorder. In: *Psychiatric Clinics of North America: Borderline personality disorder,* **23**(1), 151–167.

Clients' perspective

Haswell, D., Graham, M. (1996) Self-inflicted injuries: challenging knowledge, skill and compassion. *Canadian Family Physician,* **42**, 1756–1764.

Leibenluft, E., Gardner, D., Cowdry, R. (1987) The inner experiences of the borderline self-mutilator. *Journal of Personality Disorders,* **1**, 317–324.

Williams, L. (1998) A "classic" case of borderline personality disorder. *Psychiatric Services,* **49**, 173–174.

Hospitalization

Breeze, J.A., Repper, J. (1998) Struggling for control: the care experiences of "difficult" patients in mental health services. *Journal of Advanced Nursing,* **28**, 1301–1311.

Dawson, D., MacMillan, H. (1993) Inpatient treatment. Chapter 7 in: *Relationship management of the borderline patient: from understanding to treatment.* Brunner/Mazel, New York.

Nehls, N. (1994) Brief hospital treatment plans; innovations in practice and research. *Issues in Mental Health Nursing,* **15**, 1–15.

Nehls, N. (1994) Brief hospital treatment plans for persons with borderline personality disorder: perspectives of inpatient psychiatric nurses and community mental health centre clinicians. *Archives of Psychiatric Nursing*, **8**, 303–311.

O'Brien, L. (1998) Inpatient nursing care of patients with borderline personality disorder: a review of the literature. *Australian and New Zealand Journal of Mental Health Nursing*, **7**, 172–183.

Self-harm

Connors, R. (1996) Self injury in trauma survivors: 1. functions and meanings. *American Journal of Orthopsychiatry*, **66**, 197–206.

Connors, R. (1996) Self injury in trauma survivors: 2. levels of clinical response. *American Journal of Orthopsychiatry*, **66**, 207–216.

Substance use

Verhuel, R., van den Brink, W. (2000) The role of personality pathology in the aetiology and treatment of substance use disorders. *Current Opinion in Psychiatry*, **13**, 163–169.

Medicolegal

Fine, M., Sansone, R. (1990) Dilemmas in the management of suicidal behaviour in individuals with borderline personality disorder. *American Journal of Psychotherapy*, **44**, 160–171.

Guthcil, T.G. (1985) Medicolegal pitfalls in the treatment of borderline patients. *American Journal of Psychiatry*, **142**, 9–14.

Gutheil, T.G., Gabbard, G.D. (1993) The concept of boundaries in clinical practice: theoretical and risk management decisions. *American Journal of Psychiatry*, **150**, 188–196.

Maltsberger, J. (1994) Calculated risks in the treatment of intractably suicidal patients. *Psychiatry*, **57**, 199–212.

Stone, M. (1993) Paradoxes in the management of suicidality in borderline patients. *American Journal of Psychotherapy*, **47**, 255–272.

Relatives and friends

Gunderson, J.G., Berkowitz, C., Ruiz-Sancho, A. (1997) Families of borderline patients: A psychoeducational approach. *Bulletin of the Menninger Clinic*, **61**, 446–457.

Gunderson, J.G. (1997) Helping families with offspring having borderline personality disorder. *The Journal of the California Alliance for the Mentally Ill*, **8**, 38–40.

Hoffman, P.D. (1997) A family partnership. *The Journal of the California Alliance for the Mentally Ill,* **8,** 52–53.

Mason, P., Kreger, R. (1998) *Stop walking on eggshells: taking your life back when someone you care about has borderline personality disorder.* New Harbinger, Oakland.

Books

American Psychiatric Association. (2001) *Practice guideline for the treatment of patients with borderline personality disorder.* American Psychiatric Association, Washington DC.

Arnold, L., Magill, A. (1996) *Working with self-injury: a practical guide.* The Basement Project, Bristol.

Arnold, L., Magill, A. (1998) *The self-harm help book.* The Basement Project, Abergavenny.

Beck, A., Freeman, A. (1990) *Cognitive therapy for personality disorders.* Guilford, New York.

Benjamin, L. (1993) *Diagnosis and treatment of personality disorders.* Guilford, New York.

Briere, J. (1992) *Child abuse trauma. Theory and treatment of the lasting effects.* Sage, London.

Cauwels, J. (1992) *Imbroglio: Rising to the challenges of borderline personality disorder.* Norton, New York.

Dean, M.A. (2001) *Borderline personality disorder: the latest assessment and treatment strategies,* 2nd ed. Compact Clinicals, Kansas City.

Dawson, D., MacMillan, H.L. (1993) *Relationship management of the borderline patient: from understanding to treatment.* Brunner/Mazel, New York.

Editors. (1997) *Borderline personality disorder. The Journal of the California Alliance for the Mentally Ill,* **8**(1).

Gunderson, J.G., Gabbard, G.O. eds. (2000) *Psychotherapy for personality disorders.* Review of Psychiatry (*19*). American Psychiatric Press, Washington DC.

Gunderson, J. (2001) *Borderline personality disorder: a clinical guide.* American Psychiatric Press, Washington DC.

Herman, J. (1994) *Trauma and recovery: from domestic abuse to political terror.* Harper Collins, London.

Layden, M.A., Newman, C.F., Freeman, A., Morse, S.B. (1993) *Cognitive therapy of borderline personality disorder.* Needham Heights, Allyn and Bacon.

Linehan, M. (1993) *Cognitive behavioral treatment of borderline personality disorder.* Guilford Press, New York.

Linehan, M. (1993) *Skills training manual for treating borderline personality disorder.* Guilford Press, New York.

Links, P.S. ed. (1999) *Clinical assessment and management of severe personality disorders*. American Psychiatric Press, Washington DC.

Marziali, E., Munroe-Blum, H. (1994) *Interpersonal group psychotherapy for borderline personality disorder*. Basic Books, New York.

Mason, P., Kreger, R. (1998) *Stop walking on eggshells: taking your life back when someone you care about has borderline personality disorder*. New Harbinger, Oakland.

Meares, R. (1993) *The metaphor of play: disruption and restoration in the borderline experience*. Jason Aronson, Northvale NJ.

Miller, W.R., Rollnick, S. (1991) *Motivational interviewing – preparing people to change addictive behavior*. Guilford, New York.

Millon, T., Davis, R. (2000) *Personality disorders in modern life*. John Wiley, New York.

Milton, I., McMahon, K. eds. (1999) *Guidelines for working with serious personality disorder*. PsychOz, Melbourne.

Paris, J. ed. (1993) *Borderline personality disorder: etiology and treatment*. American Psychiatric Press, Washington DC.

Paris, J. (1994) *Borderline personality disorder: a multidimensional approach*. American Psychiatric Press, Washington DC.

Paris, J. (1998) *Working with traits: psychotherapy of personality disorders*. Jason Aronson, Northvale.

Paris, J. ed. (2000) *Borderline personality disorder*. W.B. Saunders, Psychiatric Clinics of North America Philadelphia.

Rockland, L.H. (1992) *Supportive therapy for borderline patients*. Guilford Press, New York.

Silk, K.R. ed. (1998) *Biology of personality disorders*. Review of Psychiatry, Vol 17. American Psychiatric Press, Washington DC.

Young, J.E. (1994) *Cognitive therapy for personality disorders: a schema focused approach*. Professional Resource Exchange, Sarasota.

References

Adler, G. (1993) The psychotherapy of core borderline psychopathology. *American Journal of Psychotherapy*, **47**, 194–205.

Adler, G. (1985) *Borderline psychopathology and its treatment*. New York: Aronson.

Allen, D.M. (1997) Techniques for reducing therapy-interfering behavior in patients with borderline personality disorder: similarities in four diverse treatment paradigms. *Journal of Psychotherapy Practice and Research*, **6**, 25–35.

Ames-Frankel, J., Devlin, M.J., Walsh, B.T., Strasser, T.J., Sadik, C., Oldham, J.M., Roose, S.P. (1992) Personality disorder diagnoses in patients with bulimia nervosa: clinical correlates and changes with treatment. *Journal of Clinical Psychiatry*, **53**, 90–96.

American Psychiatric Association. (1994) *Diagnostic and Statistical Manual of Mental Disorders*, Fourth edition. Washington DC: American Psychiatric Association.

American Psychiatric Association. (1998) Integrating dialectical behavior therapy into a community mental health program. *Psychiatric Services*, **49**, 1338–1340.

American Psychiatric Association. (2001) *Practice guideline for the treatment of patients with borderline personality disorder*. Washington DC: American Psychiatric Association.

Arnold, L., Magill, A. (1996) *Working with self-injury: a practical guide*. Bristol: The Basement Project.

Arnold, L., Magill, A. (1998) *The self-harm help book*. Abergavenny: The Basement Project.

Arntz, A., Dietzel, R., Dreessen, L. (1999) Assumptions in borderline personality disorder: specificity, stability and relationship with etiological factors. *Behavior Research and Therapy*, **37**, 545–557.

Barbato, N., Hafner, R.J. (1998) Comorbidity of bipolar and personality disorder. *Australian and New Zealand Journal of Psychiatry*, **32**, 276–280.

Barber, M.E., Marzuk, P.M., Leon, A.C., Portera, L. (1998) Aborted suicide attempts: a new classification of suicidal behaviour. *American Journal of Psychiatry*, **155**, 385–389.

Barley, W.D., Buie, S.E., Peterson, E.W. *et al.* (1993) Development of an inpatient cognitive behavioural treatment program for borderline personality disorder. *Journal of Personality Disorders*, **7**, 232–240.

Bateman, A., Fonagy, P. (1999) Effectiveness of partial hospitalisation in the treatment of borderline personality disorder: a randomised controlled trial. *American Journal of Psychiatry*, **156**, 1563–1569.

Bateman, A., Fonagy, P. (2001) Treatment of borderline personality disorder with psychoanalytically oriented partial hospitalisation: an 18-month follow-up. *American Journal of Psychiatry*, **158**, 36–42.

Beck, A., Freeman, A and associates. (1990) *Cognitive therapy of personality disorders*. New York: Guilford Press, pp. 186–187.

Benedetti, F., Sforzini, L., Colombo, C., Maffei, C., Smeraldi, E. (1998) Low-dose clozapine in acute and continuation treatment of severe borderline personality disorder. *Journal of Clinical Psychiatry*, **59**, 103–107.

Benjamin, L. (1993) *Diagnosis and treatment of personality disorders*. New York: Guilford.

Berelowitz, A., Tarnopolsky, M. (1993) The validity of borderline personality disorder: an updated review of recent research. In *Personality disorder reviewed*. Tyrer, P., Stein G. ed. London: Gaskell, pp. 90–112.

Bohus, M.J., Landwehrmeyer, B., Stiglmayr, C.E., Limberger, M.F., Bohme, R., Schmahl, C.G. (1999) Naltrexone in the treatment of dissociative symptoms in patients with borderline personality disorder: an open-label trial. *Journal of Clinical Psychiatry*, **60**, 598–603.

Bohus, M., Haaf, B., Stiglmayr, C., Pohl, U., Bohme, R., Linehan, M. (2000) Evaluation of inpatient dialectical-behavioral therapy for borderline personality disorder – a prospective study. *Behaviour Research and Therapy*, **38**, 875–887.

Brady, H.R., Brenner, B.M. (1998) Acute renal failure. Chapter 270 in: *Harrison's principles of internal medicine, 14th edition*. Fauci, A.S., Braunwald, E. *et al.* eds. New York: McGraw Hill 1504–1513.

Braunwald, E. (1998) Heart failure. Chapter 233 in: *Harrison's principles of internal medicine*, 14th edition. Fauci, A.S., Braunwald E *et al.* eds. New York: McGraw Hill, pp. 1287–1298.

Breeze, J.A., Repper, J. (1998) Struggling for control: the care experiences of 'difficult' patients in mental health services. *Journal of Advanced Nursing*, **28**, 1301–1311.

Briere, J. (1992) *Child abuse trauma: theory and treatment of the lasting effects*. London: Sage.

Briere, J. (1995) Substance and shadows. *New Zealand Journal of Psychotherapists Newsletter*.

Butler, R.W., Mueser, K.T., Sorock, J., Braff, D.L. (1996) Positive symptoms of psychosis in posttraumatic stress disorder. *Biological Psychiatry*, **39**, 839–844.

Cantor, C., McDermott, P. (1994) Suicide litigation; from legal to clinical wisdom. *Australian and New Zealand Journal of Psychiatry*, **28**, 431–437.

Cauwels, J. (1992) *Imbroglio: rising to the challenges of borderline personality disorder*. New York: Norton, pp. 201.

Chengappa, K.N.R., Ebeling, T., Kang, J.S., Levine, J., Parepally, H. (1999) Clozapine reduces severe self-mutilation and aggression in psychotic patients with borderline personality disorder. *Journal of Clinical Psychiatry* **60**, 477–484.

Chiesa, M., Fonagy, P. (2000) Cassel personality disorder study. Methodology and treatment effects. *British Journal of Psychiatry*, **176**, 485–491.

Clarke, M., Hafner R.J., Holme, G. (1995) Borderline personality disorder: a challenge for mental health services. *Australian and New Zealand Journal of Psychiatry*, **29**, 409–414.

Clarkin, J.F., Foelsch, P.A., Levy, K.N., Hull, J.W., Delaney, J.C., Kernberg, O.F. (2001) The development of a psychodynamic treatment for patients with borderline personality disorder: a preliminary study of personality change. *Journal of Personality Disorders*, **15**, 487–495.

Cloninger, C.R. (1998) The genetics and psychobiology of the seven-factor model of personality. Chapter 3 in: *Biology of personality disorders. Review of Psychiatry*, Vol. 17. Silk, K.R. ed. Washington DC: American Psychiatric Press, pp. 63–92.

Coccaro, E.F., Kavoussi, R.J. (1997) Fluoxetine and impulsive aggressive behavior in personality disordered subjects. *Archives of General Psychiatry*, **54**, 1081–1088.

Coccaro, E.F. (1998a) Neurotransmitter function in personality disorder. Chapter 1 in: *Biology of personality disorders. Review of Psychiatry* Vol. 17. Silk, K.R. ed. Washington DC: American Psychiatric Press, pp. 1–25.

Coccaro, E.F. (1998b) Clinical outcomes of psychopharmacologic treatment of borderline and schizotypal personality disordered subjects. *Journal of Clinical Psychiatry*, **59**(S1), 30–35.

Connors, R. (1996) Self-injury in trauma survivors: functions and meanings. *American Journal of Orthopsychiatry*, **66**, 197–206.

Crisis Recovery Service. (undated) *Philosophy and protocols for the management of self harm.* The Maudsley, The Bethlehem and Maudsley NHS Trust.

Crits-Christoff, P. (1998) Psychosocial treatments for personality disorders. Chapter 27 in: *A guide to treatments that work.* Nathan, P.E., Gorman, J.M., eds. New York: Oxford University Press, pp. 544–553.

Dawson, D.F. (1988) Treatment of the borderline patient, relationship management. *Canadian Journal of Psychiatry*, **33**, 370–374.

Dawson, D., MacMillan, H. (1993) *Relationship management of the borderline patient.* New York: Brunner/Mazel.

DiClemente, C.C. (1991) Motivational interviewing and the stages of change. Chapter 13 in *Motivational interviewing – preparing people to change addictive behavior.* New York: Guilford, pp. 51–63.

Dowson, J.H., Sussams, P., Grounds, A.T., Taylor, J. (2000) Associations of self-reported past "psychotic" phenomena with features of personality disorder. *Comprehensive Psychiatry*, **41**, 42–48.

Dubo, E.D., Zanarini, M.C., Lewis, R.E., Williams, A.A. (1997) Childhood antecedents of self-destructiveness in borderline personality disorder. *Canadian Journal of Psychiatry*, **42**, 63–69.

Dulit, R.A., Fyer, M.R., Haas, G.L., Sullivan, T., Frances, A.J. (1990) Substance use in borderline personality disorder. *American Journal of Psychiatry*, **147**, 1002–1007.

Evans, K., Tyrer, P., Catalan, J. *et al.* (1999) Manual assisted cognitive-behavior therapy (MACT): a randomised controlled trial of a brief intervention with bibliography in the treatment of deliberate self-harm. *Psychological Medicine*, **29**, 19–25.

Everett, B., Nelson, A. (1992) We're not cases and you're not managers: an account of a client-professional partnership developed in response to the "borderline" diagnosis. *Psychosocial Rehabilitation Journal*, **15**, 49–60.

Figueroa, E., Silk, K. (1997) Biological implications of childhood sexual abuse in borderline personality disorder. *Journal of Personality Disorders*, **11**, 71–92.

Fine, M.A., Sansone, R.A. (1990) Dilemmas in the management of suicidal behavior in individuals with borderline personality disorder. *American Journal of Psychotherapy*, **44**, 160–171.

Fraser, K., Gallop, R. (1993) Nurses' confirming/disconfirming responses to patients diagnosed with borderline personality disorder. *Archives of Psychiatric Nursing*, **7**, 336–341.

Gabbard, O.G., Lazar, S.G., Hornberger, J., Spiegel, D. (1997) The economic impact of psychotherapy: a review. *American Journal of Psychiatry*, **154**, 147–155.

Gabbard, G.O. (2000). Combining medication with psychotherapy in the treatment of personality disorders. Chapter 3 in: *Review of Psychiatry* 19(3). Gunderson, J.G., Gabbbard, G.O. eds. Washington DC: American Psychiatric Press, pp. 65–94.

Gallop, R., Lancee, W.J., Garfinkel, P. (1989) How nursing staff respond to the label "borderline personality disorder". *Hospital and Community Psychiatry*, **40**, 815–819.

Gardner, D., Lucas, P.B., Cowdrey, R.W. (1987) Soft sign neurological abnormalities in borderline personality disorder and normal control subjects. *Journal of Nervous and Mental Disease*, **175**, 177–180.

Gardner, D.L., Cowdrey, R.W. (1986) Positive effects of carbamazepine on behavioral dyscontrol in borderline personality disorder. *American Journal of Psychiatry*, **143**, 519–522.

Geller, J. (1993) Treating revolving-door patients who have "hospitalphilia": compassion, coercion and commonsense. *Hospital and Community Psychiatry*, **44**, 141–146.

Grilo, C.M., Martino, S., Walker, M.L., Becker, D.F., Edell, W.S., McGlashan, T.H. (1997) Controlled study of psychiatric comorbidity in psychiatrically hospitalized young adults with substance use disorders. *American Journal of Psychiatry*, **154**, 1305–1307.

Gunderson, J.G. (1984) *Borderline personality disorder*. Washington DC. American Psychiatric Press.

Gunderson, J.G., Zanarini, M.C. (1987) Current overview of the borderline diagnosis. *Journal of Clinical Psychiatry*, **48S**, 5–11.

Gunderson, J.G. (1996) The borderline patient's intolerance of aloneness: insecure attachments and therapists' availability. *American Journal of Psychiatry*, **153**, 531–546.

Gunderson, J.G., Berkowitz, C., Ruiz-Sancho, A. (1997) Families of borderline patients: A psychoeducational approach. *Bulletin of the Menninger Clinic*, **61**, 446–457.

Gunderson, J. (1999) *International Society for the Study of Personality Disorders: 6th International Congress on the Disorders of Personality*. Geneva.

Gunderson, J. (2001) *Borderline personality disorder: a clinical guide*. Washington DC: American Psychiatric Press.

Gurvits, I.G., Koenigsberg, H.W., Siever., L.J. (2000) Neurotransmitter dysfunction in patients with borderline personality disorder. *Psychiatric Clinics of North America: borderline personality disorder*, **23**(1), 27–40.

Gutheil, T.G. (1985) The medicolegal pitfalls in the treatment of borderline patients. *American Journal of Psychiatry*, **142**, 9–14.

Gutheil, T.G. (1998) Liability in psychopharmacology. (audiotape) *Audio-Digest Psychiatry* 27(10).

Hafner, J.R., Holme G. (1996) The influence of a therapeutic community on psychiatric disorder. *Journal of Clinical Psychology*, **52**, 461–468.

Hamner, M.B., Frueh, C., Ulmer, H.G., Arana, G.W. (1999) Psychotic features and illness severity in combat veterans with chronic posttraumatic stress disorder. *Biological Psychiatry*, **45**, 846–852.

Haswell, D., Graham, M. (1996) Self-inflicted injuries: challenging knowledge, skill and compassion. *Canadian Family Physician*, **42**, 1756–1764.

Hawton, K., Arensman, E., Townsend, E *et al.* (1998) Deliberate self-harm: systematic review of efficacy of psychosocial and pharmacological treatments in preventing repetition. *British Medical Journal*, **317**, 441–447.

Herman, J., Perry, C., van der Kolk, B. (1989) Childhood trauma in borderline personality disorder. *American Journal of Psychiatry*, **146**, 490–495.

Herman, J. (1992) *Trauma and Recovery: from domestic abuse to political terror*. London: Harper Collins.

Hirschfield, R.M.A. (1997) Pharmacotherapy of borderline personality disorder. *Journal of Clinical Psychiatry*, **58S**, 48–52.

Hoffman, P.D. (1997) A family partnership. *The Journal of the California Alliance for the Mentally Ill*, **8**, 52–53.

Hollander, E. (1999) Managing aggressive behavior in patients with obsessive-compulsive disorder and borderline personality disorder. *Journal of Clinical Psychiatry*, **60**(S15), 38–44.

Hollander, E., Allen, A., Prieto-Lopez, R., Bienstock, C.A., Grossman, R., Siever, L.J., Mekatz, L., Stein, D.J. (2001) A preliminary double-blind, placebo-controlled trial of divalproex sodium in borderline personality disorder. *Journal of Clinical Psychiatry*, **62**, 199–203.

Holmes, J. (1995) Supportive psychotherapy: the search for positive meanings. *British Journal of Psychiatry*, **167**, 439–445.

Hurt, S.W., Clarkin, J.F., Munroe-Blum, H., Marziali, E.A. (1992) Borderline behavior clusters and different treatment approaches. In: *Borderline personality disorder: clinical and empirical perspectives*. Clarkin, J.F., Marziali, E.A., Munroe-Blum H. eds. New York: Guilford Press, pp. 199–219.

Ivezic, S., Oruc, L., Bell, P. (1999) Psychotic symptoms in post-traumatic stress disorder. *Military Medicine*, **164**, 73–75.

Jackson, W. (1999) A personalised client's perspective of mental health treatment. *Presented at the 2nd National Conference on borderline personality disorder*, Wellington.

Kavoussi, R.J., Coccaro, E.F. (1998) Divalproex sodium for impulsive aggressive behavior in patients with personality disorder. *Journal of Clinical Psychiatry*, **59**, 676–680.

Kernberg, O.F. (1975) *Borderline conditions and pathological narcissism*. New York: Aronson.

Kjelsberg, E., Eikeseth, P.H., Dahl, A.A. (1991) Suicide in borderline patients – predictive factors. *Acta Psychiatrica Scandinavica*, **84**, 283–287.

Knutson, B., Wolkowitz, O.M., Cole, S.W., Chan, T., Moore, E.A., Johnson R.C. *et al.* (1998) Selective alteration of personality and social behavior by serotonergic intervention. *American Journal of Psychiatry*, **155**, 373–379.

Kohut, H. (1977) *The restoration of the self*. New York: International Universities Press.

Koons, C.R., Robins, C.J., Tweed, I.L., Lynch, T.R., Gonzalez, A.M., Morse, J.Q. *et al.* (2001) Efficacy of dialectical behaviour therapy in women veterans with borderline personality disorder. *Behavior Therapy*, **32**, 371–390.

Krawitz, R. (1997a) Borderline personality disorder: mental health resource use and associated funding and service delivery considerations. *Document* for *Health Waikato*.

Krawitz, R. (1997b) A prospective psychotherapy outcome study. *Australian and New Zealand Journal of Psychiatry*, **31**, 465–473.

Krawitz, R., Watson, C. (1999) *Borderline personality disorder: pathways to effective service delivery and clinical treatment options*. Wellington: Mental Health Commission, Occasional publications no. 2.

Kroll, J. (1993) *PTSD/Borderlines in therapy*. New York: Norton, p. 137.

Lancee, W.J., Gallop, R., McCay, E., Toner, B. (1995) The relationship between nurses' limit-setting style and anger in psychiatric inpatients. *Psychiatric Services* **46**, 609–613.

Laporte, L., Guttman, H. (1996) Traumatic childhood experiences as risk factors for borderline and other personality disorders. *Journal of Personality Disorders,* **10,** 247–259.

Layden, M.A., Newman, C.F., Freeman, A., Morse, S.B. (1993) *Cognitive therapy of borderline personality disorder.* Needham Heights: Allyn and Bacon.

Leibenluft, E., Gardner, D., Cowdry, R. (1987) The inner experiences of the borderline self-mutilator. *Journal of Personality Disorders,* **1,** 317–324.

Lesage, A.D., Boyer, R., Grunberg, F., Vanier, C., Morissette, R., Menard-Buteau, C., Loyer, M. (1994) Suicide and mental disorders: a case control study of young men. *American Journal of Psychiatry,* **151,** 1063–1068.

Lewis, G., Appleby, L. (1988) Personality disorder: the patients psychiatrists dislike. *British Journal of Psychiatry,* **153,** 44–49.

Lincoln, A.J., Bloom, D., Katz, M., Boksenbaum, N. (1998) Neuropsychological and neurophysiological indices of auditory processing impairment in children with multiple complex development disorder. *Journal of the American Academy of Child and Adolescent Psychiatry,* **37,** 100–112.

Linehan, M.M., Armstrong, II., Suarez, L., Allmon, D. (1991) Cognitive-behavioural treatment of chronically parasuicidal borderline patients. *Archives of General Psychiatry,* **48,** 1060–1064.

Linehan, M. (1993a) *Cognitive behavioral treatment of borderline personality disorder.* New York: Guilford Press.

Linehan, M. (1993b) *Skills training manual for treating borderline personality disorder.* New York: Guilford Press.

Linehan, M.M., Heard, H.L., Armstrong, H.E. (1993c) Naturalistic follow-up of a behavioral treatment for chronically parasuicidal borderline patients. *Archives of General Psychiatry,* **50,** 971–974.

Linehan, M.M., Heard, L. (1993d) Impact of treatment accessibility on clinical course of parasuicidal patients: reply. *Archives of General Psychiatry,* **50,** 157–158.

Linehan, M.M. (1995) *Understanding borderline personality disorder: the dialectical approach.* (Video) New York, Guilford Publications.

Linehan, M.M. (1997) Dialectical behavior therapy (DBT) for borderline personality disorder. *The Journal of the California Alliance for the Mentally Ill,* **8,** 44–46.

Linehan, M.M., Schmidt, H., Dimeff, L.A., Kanter, J., Comtois, K.A. (1999) Dialectical behavior therapy for patients with borderline personality disorder and drug dependence. *American Journal on Addiction,* **8,** 279–292.

Links, P.S., Steiner, M., Boiago, I., Irwin, D. (1990) Lithium therapy for borderline patients: preliminary findings. *Journal of Personality Disorders,* **4,** 173–181.

Links, P.S. (1993) Psychiatric rehabilitation model for borderline personality disorder. *Canadian Journal of Psychiatry,* **38,** S35–S38.

Links, P.S., Heslegrave, R., Villella, J. (1998) Psychopharmacological manage-ment of personality disorders: an outcome-focused model. Chapter 4 in: *Biology of personality disorders. Review of Psychiatry*, Vol 17. Silk, K.R. ed. Washington DC: American Psychiatric Press, pp. 93–127.

Lippman, M.C. (1998) Breast cancer. Chapter 91 in: *Harrison's principles of internal medicine*, 14th edition. Fuci, A.S., Braunwald, E. *et al.* eds. New York: McGraw Hill, pp. 562–568.

Little, J., Stephens, D. (1999) A patient-based voucher system for brief hospitalisation. *Australian and New Zealand Journal of Psychiatry*, 33, 429–432.

McGlashan, T.H. (1986) The Chestnut Lodge follow-up study: long-term outcome of borderline personalities. *Archives of General Psychiatry*, 43, 20–30.

McMahon, K., Milton, I. (1999) Behavioural modification and contracting. Chapter 6 in: *Guidelines for working with serious personality disorder*. Milton, I., McMahon, K. eds. Melbourne: PsychOz, pp. 21–23.

Maltsberger, J. (1994) Calculated risks in the treatment of intractably suicidal patients. *Psychiatry*, 57, 199–212.

Marguiles, A. (1984) Toward empathy: the uses of wonder. *American Journal of Psychiatry*, 141, 1025–1033.

Markowitz, P.J. (1995) Pharmacotherapy of impulsivity, aggression and related disorders. Chapter 16 in: *Impulsivity and agression*. Hollander, E., Stein, D. eds. Surrey: Wiley, pp. 263–287.

Masterson, J.F. (1976) *Psychotherapy of the borderline adult: a developmental approach*. New York: Brunner/Mazel.

Mason, P., Kreger, R. (1998) *Stop walking on eggshells: taking your life back when someone you care about has borderline personality disorder*. Oakland: New Harbinger.

Mazelis, R. (1997/8) SIV, reflections on healing (editorial). *The Cutting Edge: A Newsletter for Women Living with Self-Inflicted Violence*, 8(4), 1–2.

Mazelis, R. (1998) The politics of SIV: the politics of voice (editorial). *The Cutting Edge: A Newsletter for Women Living With Self-Inflicted Violence*, 9(1), 1–4.

Meares, R. (1993) *The metaphor of play: disruption and restoration in the borderline experience*. Northvale NJ: Jason Aronson.

Meares, R. (1996) The psychology of self: an update. *Australian and New Zealand Journal of Psychiatry*, 30, 312–316.

Meares, R., Stevenson, J., Comerford, A. (1999) Psychotherapy with borderline patients: a comparison between treated and untreated cohorts. *Australian and New Zealand Journal of Psychiatry*, 33, 467–472.

Miller, C.R., Eisner, W., Allport, C. (1994) Creative coping: a cognitive-behavioral group for borderline personality disorder. *Archives of Psychiatric Nursing*, 8, 280–285.

Miller, F.T., Abrams, T., Dulit, R., Fyer, M. (1993) Psychotic symptoms in patients with borderline personality disorder and concurrent Axis I disorder. *Hospital and Community Psychiatry*, 44, 59–61.

Miller, W.R. (1983) Motivational interviewing with problem drinkers. *Behavioral psychotherapy*, **11**, 147–172.

Miller, W.R., Rollnick, S. (1991) Principles of motivational interviewing. Chapter 5 in: *Motivational interviewing- preparing people to change addictive behavior.* Guilford: New York, pp. 51–63.

Millon, T. (1992) The borderline construct: introductory notes on its history, theory and empirical grounding. In: *Borderline personality disorder: clinical and empirical perspectives.* Clarkin, J.F., Marziali, E., Munroe-Blum, H., eds. New York: Guilford Press, pp. 3–26.

Millon, T. (2000) Sociocultural conceptions of the borderline personality. *Psychiatric Clinics of North America*, **23**, 123–136.

Milton, I., Banfai, A. (1999) Continuing care. Chapter 2 in: *Guidelines for working with serious personality disorder.* Milton, I., McMahon K. eds. Melbourne: PsychOz, pp. 8–12.

Milton, I., McMahon, K. (1999) Innovative group programs. Chapter 7 in: *Guidelines for working with serious personality disorder.* Milton, I., McMahon, K., eds. Melbourne: PsychOz, p. 24.

Milton, I., Dawson, K., Kazmierczak, T., Gluyas, C., McMahon, K., Zigon, I. (1999) Basic principles for understanding serious personality disorder. Chapter 1 in: *Guidelines for working with serious personality disorder.* Milton, I., McMahon, K., eds. Melbourne: PsychOz, pp. 1–7.

Ministry of Health. (1998) *Guidelines for clinical risk assessment and management in mental health services.* Wellington: Ministry of Health.

Morton, J., Buckingham, B. (1994) Service options for clients with severe or borderline personality disorders. *Document of Psychiatric Services Branch, Dept. of Health and Community Services*, Victoria.

Munroe-Blum, H., Marziali, E. (1995) A controlled trial of short term group treatment for borderline personality disorder. *Journal of Personality Disorders*, **9**, 190–198.

Nehls, N., Diamond, R.J. (1993) Developing a systems approach to caring for persons with borderline personality disorder. *Community Mental Health Journal*, **29**, 161–172.

Nehls, N. (1994) Brief hospital treatment plans: innovations in practice and research. *Issues in Mental Health Nursing*, **15**, 1–15.

NZAP (1997) New Zealand Association of Psychotherapists supervision guidelines. In: *Information for members and applicants.*

O'Brien, L., Flote, J. (1997) Providing nursing care for a patient with borderline personality disorder on an acute inpatient unit: a phenomenological study. *Australian and New Zealand Journal of Mental Health Nursing*, **6**, 137–147.

O'Brien, L. (1998) Inpatient nursing care of patients with borderline personality disorder: a review of the literature. *Australian and New Zealand Journal of Mental Health Nursing*, **7**, 172–183.

O'Connell, R.A., Mayo, J.A., Sciutto, M.S. (1991) PDQ-R personality disorders in bipolar patients. *Journal of Affective Disorders*, **23**, 217–221.

Ogata, S.N., Silk, K.R., Goodrich, S., Lohr, N.E., Westen, D., Hill, E.M. (1990) Childhood sexual and physical abuse in adults with borderline personality disorder. *American Journal of Psychiatry*, **147**, 1008–1013.

O'Leary, K.M. (2000). Neuropsychological testing results. *Psychiatric Clinics of North America: borderline personality disorder*, **23**(1), 42–60.

Oldham, J.M. (1997) Borderline personality disorder: the treatment dilemma. *The Journal of the California Alliance for the Mentally Ill*, **8**, 13–15.

Oquendo, M.A., Mann, J. (2000) The biology of impuslivity and suicidality. *Psychiatric Clinics of North America: borderline personality disorder*, **23**(1), 11–25.

Owen, M. (1998) Organisational issues in the treatment of people with borderline personality disorder. Paper presented at the *1st National Gathering on Borderline Personality Disorder*. Auckland.

Paris, J., Brown, R., Nowlis, D. (1987) Long-term follow-up of borderline patients in a general hospital. *Comprehensive Psychiatry*, **28**, 530–535.

Paris, J. (1992) Social risk factors for borderline personality disorder: a review and hypothesis. *Canadian Journal of Psychiatry*, **37**, 510–515.

Paris J. (1993) Management of acute and chronic suicidality in patients with borderline personality disorder. Chapter 17 in: *Borderline personality disorder: etiology and treatment*. Paris J. ed. Washington DC: American Psychiatric Press.

Paris, J. (1996) Cultural factors in the emergence of borderline pathology. *Psychiatry*, **59**, 185–192.

Paris, J. (1997) Borderline personality disorder: what is it? what causes it? how can we treat it? *The Journal of the California Alliance for the Mentally Ill*, **8**, 5–6.

Paris, J. (1998) Significance of biological research for a biopsychosocial model of the personality disorders. In: *Biology of personality disorders. Review of Psychiatry*, Vol 17. Silk, K.R. ed. Washington DC: American Psychiatric Press, pp. 129–148.

Paris, J., Zweig-Frank, H. (2001) A 27-year follow-up of patients with borderline personality disorder. *Comprehensive Psychiatry*, **42**, 482–487.

Paris, J. (2002) Commentary on the American Psychiatric Association guidelines for the treatment of borderline personality disorder: evidence-based psychiatry and the quality of evidence. *Journal of Personality Disorders*, **16**, 130–134.

Perry, H. (1996) Treatment options for borderline personality disorder: *Discussion paper prepared for Mental Health Services*, Waitemata Health Limited.

Pica, S., Edwards, J., Jackson, H.J., Bell, R.C., Bates, G.W., Rudd, R.P. (1990) Personality disorders in recent-onset bipolar disorder. *Comprehensive Psychiatry*, **31**, 499–510.

Pilkonis, P.A. (1997) Surveying a complex domain: research and treatment of borderline personality disorder. *The Journal of the California Alliance for the Mentally Ill*, **8**, 10–11.

Plakun, E.M., Burkhardt, P.E., Muller, J.P. (1985) 14-year follow-up of borderline and schizotypal personality disorders. *Comprehensive Psychiatry*, **26**, 448–455.

Reich, J.H., Vasile, R.G. (1993) Effect of personality disorders on the treatment outcome of Axis I conditions: an update. *Journal of Nervous and Mental Disease*, **181**, 475–484.

Robbins, J.M., Beck, P.R., Mueller, D.P., Mizener, D.A. (1988) Therapists perceptions of difficult psychiatric patients. *Journal of Nervous and Mental Disease*, **176**, 490–497.

Rockland, L.H. (1992) *Supportive therapy for borderline patients*. New York: Guilford.

Roth, A.S., Ostroff, R.B., Hoffman, R.E. (1996) Naltrexone as a treatment for repetitive self-injurious behavior: an open-label trial. *Journal of Clinical Psychiatry*, **57**, 233–237.

Runeson, B.S., Beskow, J. (1991) Borderline personality disorder in young Swedish suicides. *Journal of Nervous and Mental Disease*, **179**, 153–156.

Runeson, B.S., Beskow, J., Waern, M. (1996) The suicidal process in suicides among young people. *Acta Psychiatrica Scandinavica*, **93**, 35–42.

Ryan, K. (1997) Difference and integration in groups: 'sitting in the fire'. *Journal of the New Zealand Association of Psychotherapists*, **3**, 151–161.

Ryle, A., Golynkina, K. (2000) Effectiveness of time-limited cognitive analytic therapy of borderline personality disorder: factors associated with outcome. *British Journal of Medical Psychology*, **73**, 197–210.

Sabo, A. (1997) Etiological significance of associations between childhood trauma and borderline personality disorder: conceptual and clinical implications. *Journal of Personality Disorders*, **11**, 50–70.

Sabo, A., Gunderson, J.G., Najavits, L.M., Chauncey, D., Kisiel, C. (1995) Changes in self-destructiveness of borderline patients in psychotherapy: a prospective follow-up. *The Journal of Nervous and Mental Disease*, **183**, 370–376.

Safer, D.L., Telch, C.F., Agras, W.S. (2001) Dialectical behavior therapy for bulimia nervosa. *American Journal of Psychiatry*, **158**, 632–634.

Salkovskis, P.M., Atha, C., Storer, D. (1990) Cognitive-behavioural problem solving in the treatment of patients who repeatedly attempt suicide: a controlled trial. *British Journal of Psychiatry*, **157**, 871–876.

Salzman, C., Wolfson, A.N., Schatzberg, A., Looper, J., Henke, R., Albanese, M. et al. (1995) Effect of fluoxetine on anger in symptomatic volunteers with borderline personality disorder. *Journal of Clinical Psychopharmacology*, **15**, 23–29.

Sanderson, C., Swenson, C., Bohus, M. (2002) A critique of the American Psychiatric Association practice guideline for the treatment of patients with borderline personality disorder. *Journal of Personality Disorders*, **16**, 122–129.

Sansone, R.A., Sansone, L.A., Wiederman, M.W. (1996) Borderline personality disorder and health care utilization in a primary care setting. *Southern Medical Journal*, **89**, 1162–1165.

Sautter, F.J., Brailey, K., Uddo, M.M., Hamilton, M.F., Beard, M.G., Borges, A.H. (1999) PTSD and comorbid psychotic disorder: comparison with veterans diagnosed with PTSD or psychotic disorder. *Journal of Traumatic Stress*, **12**, 73–88.

Serban, G., Siegel, S. (1984) Response of borderline and schizotypal patients to small doses of thiothixene and haloperidol. *American Journal of Psychiatry*, **141**, 1455–1458.

Shearin, E.N., Linehan, M.M. (1992) Patient-therapist ratings and relationship to progress in dialectical behavior therapy for borderline personality disorder. *Behavior Therapy*, **23**, 730–741.

Siever, L.J. (1997) The biology of borderline personality disorder. *The Journal of the California Alliance for the Mentally Ill*, **8**, 18–19.

Silk, K. (1997) Notes on the biology of borderline personality disorder. *The Journal of the California Alliance for the Mentally Ill*, **8**, 15–17.

Sober, A.J., Koh, H.K., Tran, N.T., Washington, C.V. (1998) Melanoma and other skin cancers. Chapter 88 in: *Harrison's principles of internal medicine*, 14th edition. Fauci, A.S., Braunwald, E. *et al.* eds. New York: McGraw Hill, 543–549.

Soloff, P.H. (1997) Suicidal behavior in borderline personality disorder/ psychobiological factors. *The Journal of the California Alliance for the Mentally Ill*, **8**, 25–26.

Solloff, P.H. (2000) Psychopharmacology of borderline personality disorder. *Psychiatric Clinics of North America*, **23**(1), 169–192.

Stevenson, J., Meares, R. (1992) An outcome study of psychotherapy for patients with borderline personality disorder. *American Journal of Psychiatry*, **149**, 358–362.

Stevenson, J., Meares, R. (1999) Psychotherapy with borderline patients: a preliminary cost benefit study. *Australian and New Zealand Journal of Psychiatry*, **33**, 473–477.

Stone, M.H., Stone, D.K., Hurt, S.W. (1987) Natural history of borderline patients treated by intensive hospitalization. *Psychiatric Clinics of North America*, **10**, 185–206.

Stone, M. (1989) The course of borderline personality disorder. Chapter 6 in: *Review of Psychiatry*, Vol 8. Tasman, A., Hales, R.E., Frances, A.J., eds. Washington DC: American Psychiatric Press, pp. 103–122.

Stone, M. (1990a) *The fate of borderline patients: successful outcome and psychiatric practice.* New York: Guilford Press.

Stone, M. (1990b) Treatment of borderline patients; a pragmatic approach. *Psychiatric Clinics of North America*, **13**, 265–285.

Stone, M.H. (1993) Paradoxes in the management of suicidality in borderline patients. *American Journal of Psychotherapy*, **47**, 255–272.

Swartz, M., Blazer, D., George, L., Winfield, I. (1990) Estimating the prevalence of borderline personality disorder in the community. *Journal of Personality Disorders*, **4**, 257–272.

Tanney, B., Motto, J.A. (1990) Long-term follow up of 1570 attempted suicides. *Proceedings of the 23rd Annual Conference of the American Association of Suicidology*. New Orleans: American Association of Suicidology.

Torgerson, S. (2000) Genetics of patients with borderline personality disorder. *Psychiatric Clinics of North America: borderline personality disorder*, **23**(1), 1–9.

Trull, T.J., Sher, K.J., Minks-Brown, C., Durbin, J., Burr, R. (2000) Borderline personality disorder and substance use disorders: a review and integration. *Clinical Psychology Review*, **20**, 235–253.

Tucker, L., Bauer, S., Wagner, S., Harlam, D., Sher, I. (1987) Long-term hospital treatment of borderline patients: a descriptive outcome study. *American Journal of Psychiatry*, **144**, 1443–1448.

Turner, R.M. (2000) Naturalistic evaluation of dialectical behavior therapy-oriented treatment for borderline personality disorder. *Cognitive and Behavioral Practice*, **7**, 413–419.

Tyrer, P. (2002) Practice guideline for the treatment of borderline personality disorder: a bridge too far. *Journal of Personality Disorders*, **16**, 113–118.

Vaglum, P., Friis, S., Irion, T. *et al.* (1990) Treatment response of severe and non severe personality disorders in a therapeutic community day unit. *Journal of Personality Disorders*, **4**, 161–172.

Van Reekum, R. (1993) Acquired and developmental brain dysfunction in borderline personality disorder. *Canadian Journal of Psychiatry*, **38**, S4–S10.

Van Reekum, R., Links, P.S., Finlayson, A.J. *et al.* (1996) Repeat neurobehavioral study of borderline personality disorder. *Journal of Psychiatry and Neuroscience*, **21**, 13–20.

Verhuel, R., Hartgers, C., van den Brink, W., Koeter, M.W.J. (1998) The effect of sampling, diagnostic criteria and assessment procedures on the observed prevalence of DSM-III-R personality disorders among treated alcoholics. *Journal of Studies on Alcohol*, **59**, 227–236.

Verkes, R.J., Van der Mast, R.C., Hengeveld, M.W., Tuyl, J.P., Zwinderman, A.H., Van Kempen, G.M.J. (1998) Reduction by paroxetine of suicidal behavior in patients with repeated suicide attempts but not major depression. *American Journal of Psychiatry*, **155**, 543–547.

Widiger, T.A., Frances, A.J. (1989) Epidemiology, diagnosis and comorbidity of borderline personality disorder. In: *Review of psychiatry*. Tasman, A., Hales, R.E., Frances, A.J., eds. Washington DC: American Psychiatric Press.

Wildgoose, A., Clarke, S., Waller G. (2001) Treating personality fragmentation and dissociation in borderline personality disorder: a pilot study of the impact of cognitive analytic therapy. *British Journal of Medical Psychology*, **74**, 47–55.

Williams, L. (1998) A "classic" case of borderline personality disorder. *Psychiatric Services*, **49**, 173–174.

Woo-Ming, A.M., Siever, L.J. (1998) Psychopharmacological treatment of personality disorders. Chapter 28 in: *A guide to treatments that work*. Nathan, P.E., Gorman, J.M., eds. New York: Oxford University Press, pp. 544–553.

Young, J.E. (1994) *Cognitive therapy for personality disorders: a schema focused approach*. Sarasota: Professional Resource Exchange.

Young, J. (1996a) Schema-focused therapy for borderline patients. (audiotape) *Audio-Digest Psychiatry*, **25**(18).

Young, J. (1996b) Schema-focused therapy for borderline patients. (audiotape) *Audio-Digest Psychiatry*, **25**(19).

Young, J. (1997) Schema-focused therapy for borderline patients. *http://home.sprynet.com/sprynet/schema*

Zanarini, M.C., Frankenburg, F.R. (1997) Pathways to the development of borderline personality disorder. *Journal of Personality Disorders*, **11**, 93–104.

Zanarini, M.C., Williams, A.A., Lewis, R.E. *et al.* (1997) Reported pathological childhood experiences associated with the development of borderline personality disorder. *American Journal of Psychiatry*, **154**, 1101–1106.

Zanarini, M.C., Frankenberg, F.R., Dubo, E.D. *et al.* (1998) Axis II comorbidity of borderline personality disorder. *Comprehensive Psychiatry*, **39**, 296–302.

Zanarini, M.C., Frankenburg, F.R., Reich, B., Marino, M.F., Haynes, M.C., Gunderson, J.G. (1999) Violence in the lives of adult borderline patients. *Journal of Nervous and Mental Disease*, **187**, 65–71.

Zanarini, M.C., Ruser, T., Frankenberg, F.R., Hennen, J. (2000) The dissociative experiences of borderline patients. *Comprehensive Psychiatry*, **41**, 223–227.

Zanarini, M.C. (2000) Childhood experiences associated with the development of borderline personality disorder. *Psychiatric Clinics of North America*, **23**(1), 89–101.

Zanarini, M.C., Frankenburg, F.R. (2001) Olanzapine treatment of female borderline personality disorder patients: a double-blind, placebo-controlled trial. *Journal of Clinical Psychiatry*, **62**, 849–854.

Index